Atlas of Clinical Dermatopathology

Atlas of Clinical Dermatopathology

Infectious and Parasitic Dermatoses

Editor-in-Chief

Günter Burg MD

Department of Dermatology
University of Zurich
Zurich
Switzerland

Associate Editors

Heinz Kutzner MD

Department of Dermatology
Institute of Dermatopathology
Friedrichshafen
Germany

Werner Kempf MD

Kempf und Pfaltz Histologische Diagnostik, Zurich, Switzerland
Department of Dermatology
University of Zurich
Zurich
Switzerland

Josef Feit MD, PhD

Department of Pathology
University of Ostrava
Czech Republic

Omar Sangueza MD

Departments of Pathology and Dermatology
Wake Forest School of Medicine
Winston-Salem
NC, USA

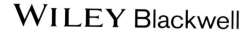

Registered Office(s)
John Wiley & Sons, Inc., 111 River Street, Hoboken, NJ 07030, United States
John Wiley & Sons Ltd, The Atrium, Southern Gate, Chichester, West Sussex, PO19 8SQ, United Kingdom

Editorial Office
9600 Garsington Road, Oxford, OX4 2DQ, United Kingdom

For details of our global editorial offices, customer services, and more information about Wiley products visit us at www.wiley.com.

Wiley also publishes its books in a variety of electronic formats and by print-on-demand. Some content that appears in standard print versions of this book may not be available in other formats.

Library of Congress Cataloging-in-Publication Data

Names: Burg, Günter, author. | Kutzner, Heinz, author. | Kempf, Werner, author. | Feit, Josef, author. | Sangueza, Omar P., author.
Title: Atlas of clinical dermatopathology : infectious and parasitic dermatoses / Editor-in-chief Günter Burg ; associate editors, Heinz Kutzner, Werner Kempf, Josef Feit, Omar Sangueza.
Description: Hoboken, NJ : Wiley-Blackwell, 2021. | Includes bibliographical references and index.
Identifiers: LCCN 2020028076 (print) | LCCN 2020028077 (ebook) | ISBN 9781119647065 (hardback) | ISBN 9781119647089 (adobe pdf) | ISBN 9781119647058 (epub)
Subjects: MESH: Skin Diseases, Infectious | Atlas
Classification: LCC RL201 (print) | LCC RL201 (ebook) | NLM WR 17 | DDC 616.5/2–dc23
LC record available at https://lccn.loc.gov/2020028076
LC ebook record available at https://lccn.loc.gov/2020028077

Cover Design: Wiley
Cover Images: © Günter Burg, © Heinz Kutzner, © Werner Kempf

Set in 10/13pt Meridien by SPi Global, Pondicherry, India

Printed and bound in Singapore by Markono Print Media Pte Ltd

10 9 8 7 6 5 4 3 2 1

To our families and teachers

Contents

Foreword   xi
Acknowledgments   xiii

1   BACTERIAL INFECTIONS   1
   1.1 Staphylococcal and
       Streptococcal Infections   2
      1.1.1   Impetigo Contagiosa   2
      1.1.2   Ostiofolliculitis (Bockardt)   4
      1.1.3   Pseudomonas (Gram-Negative) Folliculitis (Whirlpool/Hot Tub Dermatitis)   5
      1.1.4   Perianal Streptococcal Dermatitis   6
      1.1.5   Differential Diagnosis: Acne Papulopustulosa   7
      1.1.6   Differential Diagnosis: Pseudofolliculitis Barbae   8
      1.1.7   Ecthyma Gangrenosum   8
      1.1.8   Abscess   10
      1.1.9   Furuncle   11
      1.1.10 Carbuncle   12
      1.1.11 Erysipelas (Cellulitis)   13
      1.1.12 Phlegmon   15
      1.1.13 Necrotizing Fasciitis (Streptococcal Gangrene)°   17
      1.1.14 Hidradenitis Suppurativa (Acne Inversa)   17
   1.2 Other Bacterial Infections:
       Corynebacteria   18
      1.2.1   Erythrasma   18
      1.2.2   Pitted Keratolysis (Keratoma Sulcatum)   19
      1.2.3   Trichobacteriosis (Trichomycosis) Palmellina   20
      1.2.4   Erysipeloid   21
      1.2.5   Anthrax   22
      1.2.6   Nocardiosis   23
      1.2.7   Rhinoscleroma   24
   1.3 Rochalimaea/Bartonellae   25
      1.3.1   Bacillary Angiomatosis and Cat Scratch Disease   25
      1.3.2   Verruga Peruana   27
      1.3.3   Differential Diagnosis: Pyogenic Granuloma (Lobular Capillary Hemangioma; Botryomycosis)   28

   1.4 Mycobacterial Infections   29
      1.4.1   Tuberculosis Cutis   29
        1.4.1.1 Primary Tuberculosis of the Skin   30
        1.4.1.2 BCG Vaccination Granuloma   30
        1.4.1.3 Differential Diagnosis: Lupus Miliaris Disseminatus Faciei (LMDF)   31
        1.4.1.4 Lupus Vulgaris (LV)   32
        1.4.1.5 Variant: Tuberculosis (Lupus) Cutis Verrucosa   34
        1.4.1.6 Variant: Tuberculosis Cutis Colliquativa (Scrofuloderma)   35
        1.4.1.7 Lichen Scrofulosorum (Tuberculosis Cutis Lichenoides)   36
        1.4.1.8 Papulonecrotic Tuberculid   37
        1.4.1.9 Erythema Induratum Bazin   38
      1.4.2   Atypical Mycobacteriosis: Fish Tank (Swimming Pool) Granuloma   39
      1.4.3   Leprosy (Hansen Disease)   40
        1.4.3.1 Tuberculoid Leprosy   41
        1.4.3.2 Borderline Leprosy   42
        1.4.3.3 Lepromatous Leprosy   43
        1.4.3.4 Variant: Histoid Lepromatous   45
        1.4.3.5 Variant: Erythema Nodosum Leprosum   46
      1.4.4   Buruli Ulcer   47
   1.5 Actinomycosis   48

1.6   **Borrelia Infections**
       (Lyme Disease)   **49**
       1.6.1 Variant: Erythema
              (Chronicum) Migrans
              (ECM) (Stage I)   50
       1.6.2 Variant: Lymphadenosis
              Cutis Benigna
              (Pseudolymphoma,
              Lymphocytoma Cutis)
              (Stage I)   52
       1.6.3 Variant: Morphea/
              Scleroderma-Like Lesions
              (Stage II)   55
       1.6.4 Variant: Acrodermatitis
              Chronica Atrophicans
              (Stage III)   56
       1.6.5 Variant: Juxta-Articular
              Fibrous Nodules
              in Acrodermatitis
              Chronica Atrophicans
              (Stage III)   58
       1.6.6 Differential Diagnosis:
              Actinic Reticuloid°   59
1.7   **Venereal Diseases**   **59**
       1.7.1 Gonorrhea   59
       1.7.2 Syphilis, Chancre   60
              1.7.2.1 Stage I   60
              1.7.2.2 Stage II   61
              1.7.2.3 Stage III°   62
       1.7.3 Ulcus Molle (Chancroid)   63
       1.7.4 Granuloma Inguinale
              (Donovanosis; Granuloma
              Venereum)   63
       1.7.5 Lymphogranuloma
              Inguinale
              (Lymphogranuloma
              Venereum; Duran-
              Nicolas–Favre Disease)   64
1.8   **Rickettsial Infections**   **65**
1.9   **Dermatoses Associated**
       with Bacterial Infections   **66**
       1.9.1 Staphylococcal Scalded
              Skin Syndrome (SSSS)   66
       1.9.2 Differential Diagnosis:
              Toxic Epidermal
              Necrolysis (TEN)   67
1.10   **Dermatoses Mimicking**
       Bacterial Infections   **68**
       1.10.1 Pyoderma
              Gangrenosum   68
       1.10.2 Infantile Acropustulosis   70
       1.10.3 Acute Generalized
              Exanthematous
              Pustulosis (AGEP)   71

       1.10.4 Psoriasis Pustulosa   72
       1.10.5 Localized Neutrophilic
              Eccrine Hidradenitis
              Associated with
              Mitoxantrone Treatment   73
       1.10.6 Erosive Pustular Dermatitis
              (Pustular Ulcerative
              Dermatosis) of the Scalp   74
2   **FUNGAL INFECTIONS**   **77**
2.1   **Superficial Cutaneous**
       Fungal Infections   **78**
       2.1.1 Variants: Tinea Corporis;
              Tinea Faciei   79
       2.1.2 Variants: Tinea Barbae;
              Tinea Capitis
              (Trichophytia)   80
       2.1.3 Granuloma Trichophyticum
              (Majocchi's Granuloma)   82
       2.1.4 Candidiasis (Moniliasis)   83
       2.1.5 Candida Tropicalis
              and Candida Lipolytica   85
       2.1.6 Pityriasis (Tinea) Versicolor 86
       2.1.7 Variant: Malassezia
              (Pityrosporum) Folliculitis   87
       2.1.8 Differential Diagnosis:
              Seborrheic Dermatitis   88
       2.1.9 Tinea Nigra   89
       2.1.10 Piedra (Trichomycosis
              Nodosa Alba and Nigra)°   90
2.2   **Subcutaneous Mycoses**   **90**
       2.2.1 Sporotrichosis   90
       2.2.2 Mycetoma (Madura Foot)   91
       2.2.3 Chromo(blasto)mycosis
              (Dermatitis Verrucosa)   92
2.3   **Systemic Mycoses (Deep**
       Fungal Infections)   **93**
       2.3.1 Cryptococcosis (Torulosis,
              European Blastomycosis)   94
       2.3.2 North American
              Blastomycosis
              (Blastomycosis, Chicago
              Disease)   96
       2.3.3 Lobomycosis (Lobo Disease,
              Keloidal Blastomycosis,
              Blastomycoid Granuloma) 98
       2.3.4 Histoplasmosis   99
       2.3.5 Coccidioidomycosis
              (Desert or Valley Fever,
              San Joaquin Fever)   100
       2.3.6 Paracoccidioidomycosis
              (South American
              Blastomycosis)   101
       2.3.7 Emmonsiosis   102

2.4 **Opportunistic Fungal Infections** **103**
   2.4.1 Aspergillosis (Alternaria) 103
   2.4.2 Zygomycosis
      (Mucormycosis;
      Phycomycosis) 104
   2.4.3 Hyalohyphomycosis 105
   2.4.4 Phaeohyphomycosis 106
   2.4.5 Protothecosis, Cutaneous 107

3 VIRAL INFECTIONS **109**
3.1 Herpes Viruses **110**
   3.1.1 Herpes Simplex
      (HSV-1, HSV-2) 110
   3.1.2 Varizella/Zoster Virus
      (VZV/HHV-3) 111
      3.1.2.1 Varicella
          (Chickenpox) 112
      3.1.2.2 Herpes Zoster
          (Shingles) 113
      3.1.2.3 Special Feature:
          Necrotizing
          (Herpes) Zoster
          Folliculitis 115
      3.1.2.4 Special Feature:
          Zoster-Associated
          Vasculitis 116
      3.1.2.5 Postherpetic
          Cutaneous
          Reactions° 117
   3.1.3 Burkitt Lymphoma;
      Epstein-Barr Virus
      (HHV-4; EBV) 117
   3.1.4 Hairy Leukoplakia
      (HHV-4; Epstein-Barr
      Virus; EBV) 118
   3.1.5 Cytomegalovirus
      (CMV; HHV-5) 119
   3.1.6 Exanthema Subitum
      (HHV-6) (Roseola
      Infantum, 6th Disease) 120
   3.1.7 Pityriasis Rosea (HHV-7) 121
   3.1.8 AIDS-Kaposi Sarcoma
      (HHV-8) 122
   3.1.9 Multicentric Castleman's
      Disease (HHV-8) 127
3.2 Human Papilloma Virus (HPV) **128**
   3.2.1 Verruca Vulgaris 129
   3.2.2 Variant: Verrucae Planae 132
   3.2.3 Variant: Condylomata
      Acuminata 133
   3.2.4 Differential Diagnosis:
      Acrokeratosis
      Verruciformis (Hopf) 134

   3.2.5 Bowenoid Papulosis 135
   3.2.6 Epidermodysplasia
      Verruciformis
      (Lewandowsky–Lutz);
      Verrucosis Generalisata 136
3.3 Viral Exanthema **137**
   3.3.1 Measles 138
3.4 Parvovirus Infections and Coxsackievirus Infections **139**
   3.4.1 Erythema Infectiosum;
      (Slapped Cheek Disease;
      Fifth Disease) 139
   3.4.2 Papular Purpuric Gloves-
      and-Socks Syndrome 140
   3.4.3 Hand-Foot-and-Mouth
      Disease (Coxsackie Virus) 141
3.5 Polyoma Virus Infections **142**
   3.5.1 Trichodysplasia
      Spinulosa 142
   3.5.2 Merkel Cell Carcinoma
      (Primary Neuroendocrine
      Carcinoma of the Skin;
      Trabecular Carcinoma
      of Toker) 144
3.6 Poxviruses **146**
   3.6.1 Orthopox Virus Infections 146
      3.6.1.1 Cowpox (Catpox) 147
      3.6.1.2 Vaccinia Inoculata 148
      3.6.1.3 Smallpox
          (Variola Vera) 148
   3.6.2 Parapox Virus Infections 149
      3.6.2.1 Ecthyma
          Contagiosum (Orf) 149
      3.6.2.2 Variant: Milker's
          Nodule 150
      3.6.2.3 Molluscum
          Contagiosum 151
3.7 Other Skin Diseases with Suspected Viral Association **152**
   3.7.1 Asymmetric Periflexural
      Exanthema of Childhood 152
   3.7.2 Eruptive
      Pseudoangiomatosis 153
   3.7.3 Gianotti–Crosti Syndrome 154
   3.7.4 Pityriasis Lichenoides 155

4 PARASITOSES **159**
4.1 Protozoan Diseases **160**
   4.1.1 Leishmaniasis 160
   4.1.2 Variant: Leishmaniasis
      Mexicana 162
   4.1.3 Amebiasis: Entamoeba
      Histolytica 163
   4.1.4 Rhinosporidiosis 164

4.2 Arthropod: *Arachnids*   **165**
  4.2.1 Mites   165
     4.2.1.1 Demodex
           Folliculorum   166
     4.2.1.2 Scabies   167
     4.2.1.3 Variant: Scabies
           Crustosa   168
     4.2.1.4 Trombidiosis
           (Harvest Mites;
           Chigger Itch)   169
  4.2.2 Spiders°   169
  4.2.3 Ticks°   170
  4.2.4 Insects   170
  4.2.5 Tungiasis (Sand Flea)   171

**5 HELMINTHIC INFECTIONS
(PARASITIC WORMS)**   **173**
**5.1 Larva Migrans (Plumber's
Itch; Creeping Eruption)**   **174**
5.2 Filariasis   **175**
**5.3 Onchocerciasis (River
Blindness)**   **176**

5.4 Cysticercosis   **177**
5.5 Sparganosis   **177**
**5.6 Schistosomiasis
(Bilharziasis)**   **178**
**5.7 Cercarial Dermatitis
(Swimmer's Itch)**   **179**
**5.8 Annelida (Ringed Worms;
Segmented Worms)°**   **180**
5.9 Hirudinea (Leeches)   **180**

6 SEPSIS   **181**
6.1 Septic Vasculitis   **182**
6.2 Bacterial Sepsis   **185**
  6.2.1 Gonococcal Sepsis   185
6.3 Fungal Sepsis   **186**
  6.3.1 Variant: Penicillium
       Marinum Sepsis   186
  6.3.2 Variant: Candida Sepsis   187
  6.3.3 Variant: Aspergillus Sepsis   187

Index   189

°no pictures

Foreword

Atlas of Clinical Dermatopathology

Vol III

Infectious and Parasitic Dermatoses

A myriad of microbes live in us, on us, and around us in a symbiotic or parasitic relationship, fighting with our local cutaneous or systemic defense mechanisms. Without claim of being comprehensive or of following standard biologic taxonomies, this third volume on clinical dermatopathology contains more than 100 infectious and parasitic dermatoses, the clinical features (CFs) and histological features (HFs) of which are described with short concise text and information in bullet-point style. They are illustrated in over 600 high-resolution pictures with annotations. A final chapter deals with sepsis.

Since CFs and HFs are nonspecific in many cases, searching for bacterial or fungal pathogens using special stains, microbiologic cultures, or PCR probes may be helpful tools in confirming the diagnosis.

Editor-in-Chief
Günter Burg

Associate Editors
Heinz Kutzner
Werner Kempf
Josef Feit
Omar Sangueza

Acknowledgments

Many of the histological images shown are taken from the *Hypertext Atlas of Dermatopathology* (https://atlases.muni.cz/) edited by Josef Feit, Hana Jedličková, Günter Burg, Luděk Matyska, Spasoje Radovanovic, Werner Kempf, Leo Schärer et al.) Computational resources for the atlases were provided by the CESNET LM2015042 and CERIT Scientific Cloud LM2015085 large research and development programs.

The chapter on leprosy (Hansen disease) was prepared in cooperation with Ram Chandra Adhikari, MD, Consultant Dermatopathologist, DISHARC Hospital, Kathmandu, Nepal.

For basic information on clinical Dermatology you may refer free of charge to the e-learning platform DOIT (Dermatology Online with Interactive Technology: https://cyberderm.net/en/home/login.html).

We are grateful to the following colleagues, who kindly have provided clinical or hstological pictures: Luis Requena, MD, Madrid/Spain; Marianne Gloor, MD, Zürich-Bülach/Switzerland; Regina Fölster-Holst, MD, Kiel, Germany.

We appreciate the language editing by Angela Niehaus, MD, and Karen Strenge, MD, Wake Forest, North Carolina, United States, and by Aravind Kannankara, United Kingdom the support of the Wiley Publishing Group and its co-workers, especially by Bhavya Boopathi.

CHAPTER 1

Bacterial Infections

CHAPTER MENU

1.1 Staphylococcal and Streptococcal Infections
  1.1.1 Impetigo Contagiosa
  1.1.2 Ostiofolliculitis (Bockardt)
  1.1.3 Pseudomonas (Gram-Negative) Folliculitis (Whirlpool/Hot Tub Dermatitis)
  1.1.4 Perianal Streptococcal Dermatitis
  1.1.5 Differential Diagnosis: Acne Papulopustulosa
  1.1.6 Differential Diagnosis: Pseudofolliculitis Barbae
  1.1.7 Ecthyma Gangrenosum
  1.1.8 Abscess
  1.1.9 Furuncle
  1.1.10 Carbuncle
  1.1.11 Erysipelas (Cellulitis)
  1.1.12 Phlegmon
  1.1.13 Necrotizing Fasciitis (Streptococcal Gangrene)°
  1.1.14 Hidradenitis Suppurativa (Acne Inversa)
1.2 Other Bacterial Infections: Corynebacteria
  1.2.1 Erythrasma
  1.2.2 Pitted Keratolysis (Keratoma Sulcatum)
  1.2.3 Trichobacteriosis (Trichomycosis) Palmellina
  1.2.4 Erysipeloid
  1.2.5 Anthrax
  1.2.6 Nocardiosis
  1.2.7 Rhinoscleroma
1.3 Rochalimaea/Bartonellae
  1.3.1 Bacillary Angiomatosis and Cat Scratch Disease
  1.3.2 Verruga Peruana
  1.3.3 Differential Diagnosis: Pyogenic Granuloma (Lobular Capillary Hemangioma; Botryomycosis)
1.4 Mycobacterial Infections
  1.4.1 Tuberculosis Cutis
  1.4.2 Atypical Mycobacteriosis: Fish Tank (Swimming Pool) Granuloma
  1.4.3 Leprosy (Hansen Disease)
  1.4.4 Buruli Ulcer
1.5 Actinomycosis

1.6 Borrelia Infections (Lyme Disease)
  1.6.1 Variant: Erythema (Chronicum) Migrans (ECM) (Stage I)
  1.6.2 Variant: Lymphadenosis Cutis Benigna (Pseudolymphoma, Lymphocytoma Cutis) (Stage I)
  1.6.3 Variant: Morphea/Scleroderma-Like Lesions (Stage II)
  1.6.4 Variant: Acrodermatitis Chronica Atrophicans (Stage III)
  1.6.5 Variant: Juxta-Articular Fibrous Nodules in Acrodermatitis Chronica Atrophicans (Stage III)
  1.6.6 Differential Diagnosis: Actinic Reticuloid°
1.7 Venereal Diseases
  1.7.1 Gonorrhea
  1.7.2 Syphilis, Chancre
  1.7.3 Ulcus Molle (Chancroid)
  1.7.4 Granuloma Inguinale (Donovanosis; Granuloma Venereum)
  1.7.5 Lymphogranuloma Inguinale (Lymphogranuloma Venereum; Duran-Nicolas–Favre Disease)
1.8 Rickettsial Infections
1.9 Dermatoses Associated with Bacterial Infections
  1.9.1 Staphylococcal Scalded Skin Syndrome (SSSS)
  1.9.2 Differential Diagnosis: Toxic Epidermal Necrolysis (TEN)
1.10 Dermatoses Mimicking Bacterial Infections
  1.10.1 Pyoderma Gangrenosum
  1.10.2 Infantile Acropustulosis
  1.10.3 Acute Generalized Exanthematous Pustulosis (AGEP)
  1.10.4 Psoriasis Pustulosa
  1.10.5 Localized Neutrophilic Eccrine Hidradenitis Associated with Mitoxantrone Treatment
  1.10.6 Erosive Pustular Dermatitis (Pustular Ulcerative Dermatosis) of the Scalp

°no pictures

Atlas of Clinical Dermatopathology: Infectious and Parasitic Dermatoses, First Edition. Günter Burg, Heinz Kutzner, Werner Kempf, Josef Feit, and Omar Sangueza.
© 2021 John Wiley & Sons Ltd. Published 2021 by John Wiley & Sons Ltd.

1.1 Staphylococcal and Streptococcal Infections

1.1.1 Impetigo Contagiosa

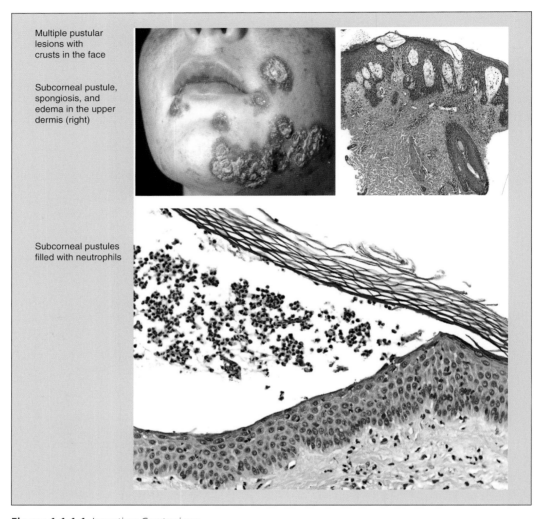

Multiple pustular
lesions with
crusts in the face

Subcorneal pustule,
spongiosis, and
edema in the upper
dermis (right)

Subcorneal pustules
filled with neutrophils

Figure 1.1.1.1 Impetigo Contagiosa.

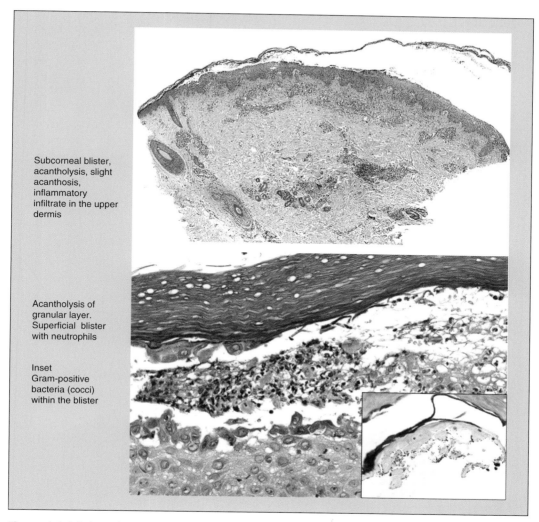

Subcorneal blister, acantholysis, slight acanthosis, inflammatory infiltrate in the upper dermis

Acantholysis of granular layer. Superficial blister with neutrophils

Inset Gram-positive bacteria (cocci) within the blister

Figure 1.1.1.2 Impetigo Contagiosa.

CF: Streptococcal infections initially induce erythematous patches with fragile subcorneal tiny vesicles, which easily rupture and develop into yellowish crusts.

Bullous lesions with thicker blister roof are usually due to staphylococcal infection.

The face and extremities of children are the most common localizations.

Impetiginization of various inflammatory skin disorders is caused by secondary infection.

HF:

- Subcorneal vesicles filled with neutrophils
- Acantholytic changes in the granular layer
- The thin roof of the pustule is often detached and replaced by necrotic crusty debris
- Neutrophil-rich lymphohistiocytic infiltrate in the upper dermis

DD: Pemphigus foliaceus (similar histology, no bacteria, positive direct immunofluorescence).

Reference

Darmstadt, G. L., & Lane, A. T. (1994). Impetigo: An overview. *Pediatr Dermatol*, **11**(4), 293–303.

Durdu, M., Baba, M., & Seckin, D. (2008). The value of Tzanck smear test in diagnosis of erosive, vesicular, bullous, and pustular skin lesions. *J Am Acad Dermatol*, **59**(6), 958–964.

1.1.2 Ostiofolliculitis (Bockardt)

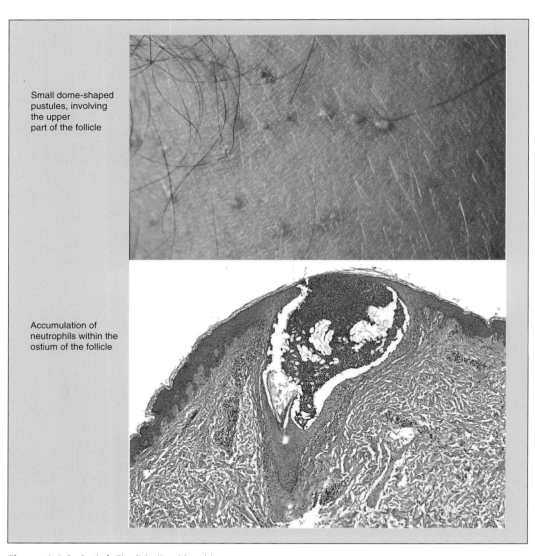

Small dome-shaped pustules, involving the upper part of the follicle

Accumulation of neutrophils within the ostium of the follicle

Figure 1.1.2 Ostiofolliculitis (Bockhardt).

Folliculitis is a general term, describing inflammatory reactions within and around follicular structures. There are many types of folliculitis, including infectious, inflammatory, mechanical, or chemical ones. In infectious folliculitis bacterial, fungal or viral agents can be involved, mostly in conjunction with predisposing factors like diabetes, atopic dermatitis, or immunodeficiencies.

Staphylococcus aureus, Streptococcus pyogenes, and *Pseudomonas aeruginosa* most commonly affect follicular structures, leading to acute superficial folliculitis, with or without deep abscess formation or chronic granulomatous inflammation. Bacterial and fungal folliculitis show similar microscopic features.

CF: Small yellow, dome-shaped pustules in a follicular distribution with the terminal or vellus hair in the center. Preferential localizations are scalp, face, and axillae.

HF: Bacterial and fungal folliculitis show similar microscopic features. Neutrophils are present in the upper part of the follicle, the infundibulum, or the subcorneal layer of the epidermis.

DD: Other forms of infectious, mechanical, or chemical folliculitis.

1.1.3 Pseudomonas (Gram-Negative) Folliculitis (Whirlpool/Hot Tub Dermatitis)

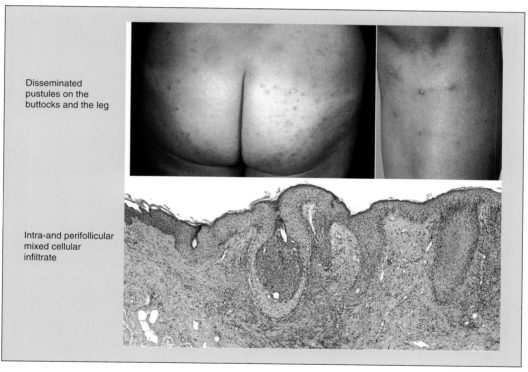

Disseminated pustules on the buttocks and the leg

Intra-and perifollicular mixed cellular infiltrate

Figure 1.1.3 Pseudomonas (Gram-Negative) Folliculitis (Whirlpool Dermatitis).

Pseudomonas aeruginosa is a gram-negative bacterium which is part of the normal flora of the large skin folds and intertriginous areas. Under special local predisposing conditions or in patients with diabetes or patients under immunosuppression, "whirlpool" or hot tub folliculitis may develop.

CF: Disseminated painful pustules, mostly at body sites covered by bathing suit.

HF:

- Follicles, with follicle walls partly ruptured
- Acneiform intra- and perifollicular inflammatory infiltrate, predominantly neutrophilic
- Plasma cells and eosinophils may be present

DD: Acne; other bacterial, fungal (pityrosporum) or viral (HIV-associated) folliculitis; demodex folliculitis.

Reference

Mazza, J., Borkin, M., Buchholz, R., & Deleo, V. (2013). Pseudomonas folliculitis contracted from rubber gloves: A public health concern. *J Am Acad Dermatol*, **69**(2), e93–94.

Yu, Y., Cheng, A. S., Wang, L., Dunne, W. M., & Bayliss, S. J. (2007). Hot tub folliculitis or hot hand-foot syndrome caused by Pseudomonas aeruginosa. *J Am Acad Dermatol*, **57**(4), 596–600.

1.1.4 Perianal Streptococcal Dermatitis

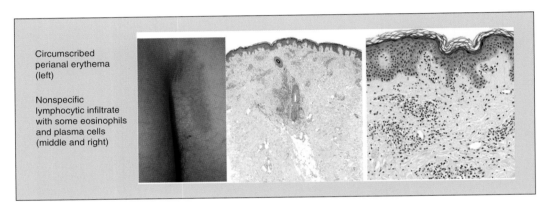

Circumscribed perianal erythema (left)

Nonspecific lymphocytic infiltrate with some eosinophils and plasma cells (middle and right)

Figure 1.1.4 Perianal Streptococcal Dermatitis.

This is caused by group B *β-hemolytic streptococci*. Similar symptoms may more frequently be caused by perianal allergic, toxic, seborrheic, or atopic dermatitis.

CF: Circumscribed pruritic eczematous erythema in the gluteal and perianal region, mostly by bacterial dissemination from the upper respiratory tract, most commonly in young children but also in adults.

HF: Variable nonspecific histologic features. Diagnosis depends on positive swab for β-hemolytic streptococci. The rationale for taking a biopsy may lie in the exclusion of other conditions (differential diagnoses; see below).

DD: Erysipelas; fungal infection; contact dermatitis; psoriasis; Langerhans cell histiocytosis; zinc deficiency/acrodermatitis enteropathica; intertrigo; lichen planus.

Reference

Kahlke, V., Jongen, J., Peleikis, H. G., & Herbst, R. A. (2013). Perianal streptococcal dermatitis in adults: Its association with pruritic anorectal diseases is mainly caused by group B Streptococci. *Colorectal Dis*, **15**(5), 602–607.

Serban, E. D. (2018). Perianal infectious dermatitis: An underdiagnosed, unremitting and stubborn condition. *World J Clin Pediatr*, **7**(4), 89–104.

1.1.5 Differential Diagnosis: Acne Papulopustulosa

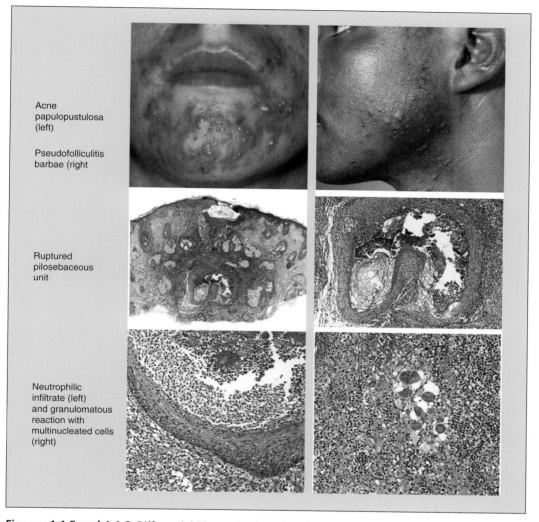

Acne
papulopustulosa
(left)

Pseudofolliculitis
barbae (right

Ruptured
pilosebaceous
unit

Neutrophilic
infiltrate (left)
and granulomatous
reaction with
multinucleated cells
(right)

Figures 1.1.5 and 1.1.6 Differential Diagnosis: Acne Papulopustulosa and Pseudofolliculitis Barbae.

CF: Papulopustular lesions, preferentially in the face during puberty and in adolescence. Various grades of severity: acne comedonica (I); acne papulopustulosa (II); acne conglobata (III).

HF (acne papulopustulosa):

• Ruptured hair follicle
• Hyperparakeratosis in the ostium and infundibular parts of the hair follicles with keratin and cellular debris

• Microorganisms (*Propionibacterium acnes* and *Staphylococcus epidermidis*) surrounded by infiltration with neutrophils
• Foreign body (granulomatous) reaction

Reference

Leyden, J. J. (1995). New understandings of the pathogenesis of acne. *J Am Acad Dermatol*, **32**(5 Pt 3), S15–25.

1.1.6 Differential Diagnosis: Pseudofolliculitis Barbae

CF: Preferentially in black people with curly hair, recurrent papular and pustular, acneiform lesions occur in the beard area, secondary to razor shaving, and in the neck, where acne keloidalis nuchae is a frequent sequela.

HF:

- Fragments of hair, penetrating into the skin
- Perifollicular and follicular inflammatory infiltrate

- Foreign body reaction with multinucleated giant cells
- Fibrosis

Reference

Perry, P. K., Cook-Bolden, F. E., Rahman, Z., Jones, E., & Taylor, S. C. (2002). Defining pseudofolliculitis barbae in 2001: A review of the literature and current trends. *J Am Acad Dermatol*, **46**(2 Suppl Understanding), S113–119.

1.1.7 Ecthyma Gangrenosum

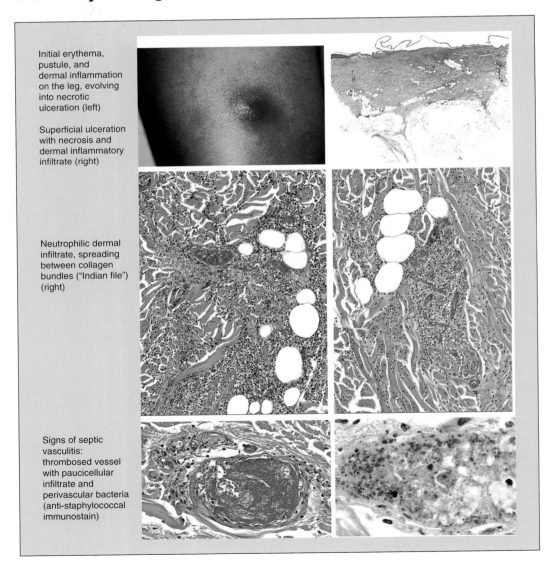

Initial erythema, pustule, and dermal inflammation on the leg, evolving into necrotic ulceration (left)

Superficial ulceration with necrosis and dermal inflammatory infiltrate (right)

Neutrophilic dermal infiltrate, spreading between collagen bundles ("Indian file") (right)

Signs of septic vasculitis: thrombosed vessel with paucicellular infiltrate and perivascular bacteria (anti-staphylococcal immunostain)

Figure 1.1.7 Ecthyma Gangrenosum.

The term *ecthyma* is used in various semantic combinations, which show different etiologies: Ecthyma simplex is a superficial ulcerating form of impetigo with "punched-out" sharp borders. Ecthyma contagiosum (orf) is caused by parapox infection (orf virus; see below).

Ecthyma gangrenosum is an ulcerative variant of septic vasculitis caused by group A streptococci or *S. aureus*. It commonly is found in tropical areas, in children, or in patients with impaired immunity.

CF: Starting with diffuse erythema, followed by massive edema, pustulation and rapid ulceration, often as sequela to minor trauma; rapid evolution into sharply circumscribed deep ulceration with distinct borders. The limbs of children (buttocks) are preferentially affected. Dissemination may occur (requiring rapid response with antibiotic treatment!). Healing with scar formation.

HF:

- Initially massive edema with subtle mixed inflammatory infiltrate
- Signs of septic vasculitis may be present (thrombosed postcapillary venules with very sparse adjacent inflammatory infiltrate)
- Gram-positive cocci, often adjacent to thrombosed vessels
- Sharply circumscribed "punched-out" deep ulceration
- Debris and necrotic material within the ulcer
- Mostly neutrophilic dermal infiltrate

DD: Ulcerating suppurative inflammation and septic vasculitis of other causes; reactive perforating dermatosis (acute prurigo).

Reference

Greene, S. L., Su, W. P., & Muller, S. A. (1984). Ecthyma gangrenosum: Report of clinical, histopathologic, and bacteriologic aspects of eight cases. *J Am Acad Dermatol*, **11**(5 Pt 1), 781–787.

1.1.8 Abscess

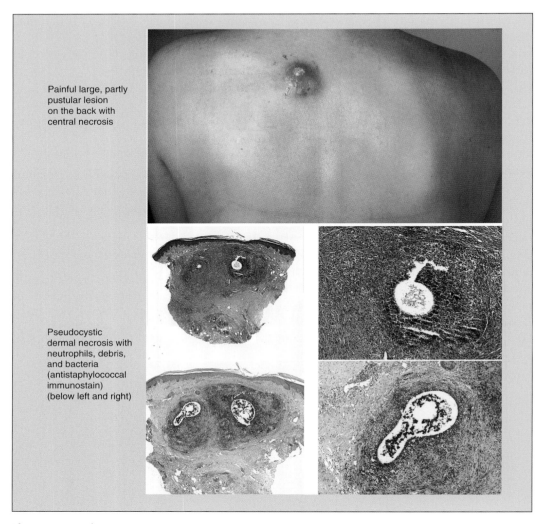

Painful large, partly pustular lesion on the back with central necrosis

Pseudocystic dermal necrosis with neutrophils, debris, and bacteria (antistaphylococcal immunostain) (below left and right)

Figure 1.1.8 Abscess.

CF: Mostly painful and highly inflamed intradermal accumulation of pus, opening and draining to the surface.

HF: Intradermal necrosis and massive suppuration with intradermal pseudocystic accumulation of neutrophils and debris.
DD: Furuncle; carbuncle; ecthyma.

1.1.9 Furuncle

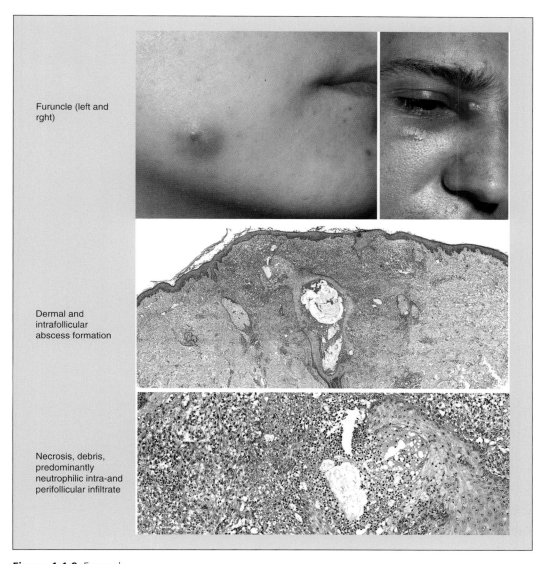

Furuncle (left and rght)

Dermal and intrafollicular abscess formation

Necrosis, debris, predominantly neutrophilic intra-and perifollicular infiltrate

Figure 1.1.9 Furuncle.

CF: Under conditions of poor hygiene or in patients with diabetes or with reduced immune status, acute deep forms of folliculitis can develop, which – depending on the size and depth – is referred to as furuncle.

HF: Deep folliculitis is usually accompanied by follicular destruction and resolves with scarring.

- Mixed inflammatory intra- and perifollicular infiltrates
- Neutrophils predominate
- Follicular rupture with abscess formation
- Granulation tissue with giant cells
- Bacterial organisms
- Necrosis
- Scarring in late lesions

DD: Abscess; carbuncle.

1.1.10 Carbuncle

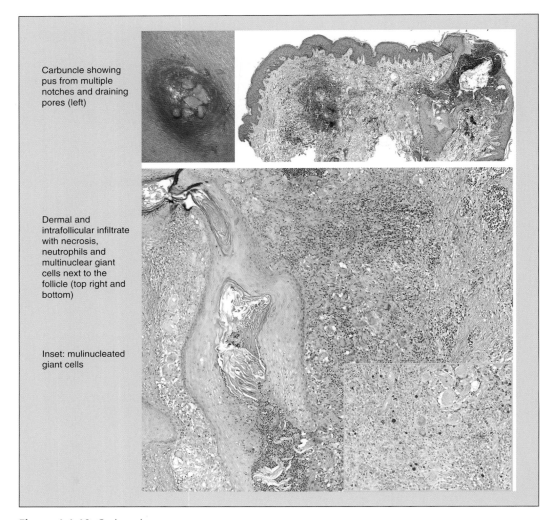

Carbuncle showing pus from multiple notches and draining pores (left)

Dermal and intrafollicular infiltrate with necrosis, neutrophils and multinuclear giant cells next to the follicle (top right and bottom)

Inset: mulinucleated giant cells

Figure 1.1.10 Carbuncle.

CF: A carbuncle comprises a large nodular furunculoid coalescing purulent lesion involving multiple follicles producing a circumscribed highly inflamed soft nodule, which extrudes pus from multiple notches and openings. Preferential localization is the trunk.
HF:

- Damage of dermal and adnexal structures
- Abscess formation and necrosis
- Granuloma formation with multinucleated giant cells
- Clusters of bacilli (Gram)
- Granulomatous reaction with multinucleated giant cells
- Resolves with scarring

1.1.11 Erysipelas (Cellulitis)

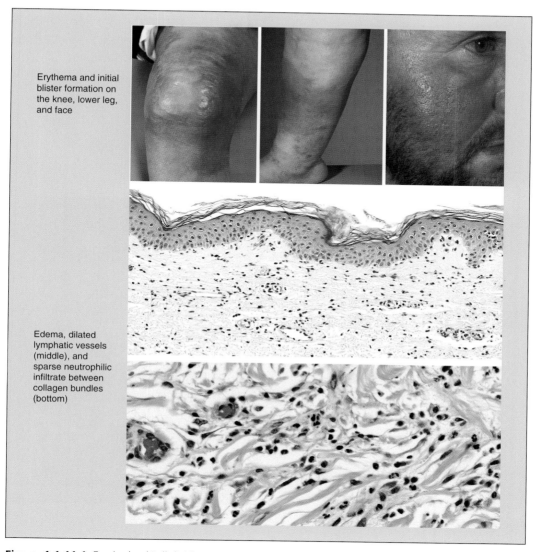

Erythema and initial blister formation on the knee, lower leg, and face

Edema, dilated lymphatic vessels (middle), and sparse neutrophilic infiltrate between collagen bundles (bottom)

Figure 1.1.11.1 Erysipelas (Cellulitis).

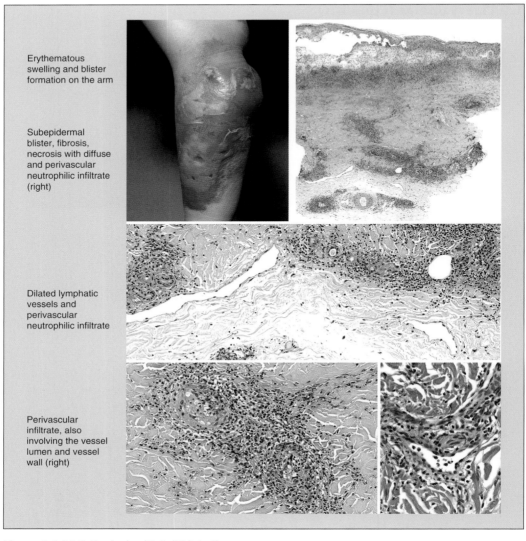

Erythematous swelling and blister formation on the arm

Subepidermal blister, fibrosis, necrosis with diffuse and perivascular neutrophilic infiltrate (right)

Dilated lymphatic vessels and perivascular neutrophilic infiltrate

Perivascular infiltrate, also involving the vessel lumen and vessel wall (right)

Figure 1.1.11.2 Erysipelas (Cellulitis), bullous.

CF: Following infection with streptococci type A via interdigital maceration or small defects, sharply demarcated peripherally spreading warm and painful erythema develops along superficial lymph vessels, preferentially on the lower legs, arms, or face. Lymphedema is a predisposing factor. Nosologic relationship exists to phlegmon and necrotizing cellulitis. Cellulitis is a maximal variant of erysipelas with dermal and subcutaneous involvement, necrosis and blister formation, which may be hemorrhagic.

Associated general symptoms are fever, chills, and swelling of the regional lymph nodes. Erysipelas has a tendency to recur.

HF:

- Dermal edema
- Dilated capillaries and lymphatic vessels
- Sparse mixed interstitial and perivascular infiltrate with neutrophils and eosinophils

- Neutrophils in vessel walls and dilated lymphatic vessels
- Occasionally subepidermal blister formation
- Fibrosis in recurrent cases

DD: Contact dermatitis, rosacea, lupus erythematosus, seborrheic dermatitis: in these conditions, fever and chills are characteristically lacking.

1.1.12 Phlegmon

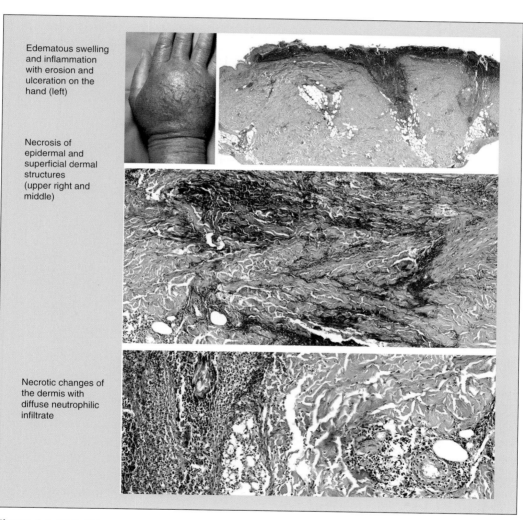

Edematous swelling and inflammation with erosion and ulceration on the hand (left)

Necrosis of epidermal and superficial dermal structures (upper right and middle)

Necrotic changes of the dermis with diffuse neutrophilic infiltrate

Figure 1.1.12.1 Phlegmon.

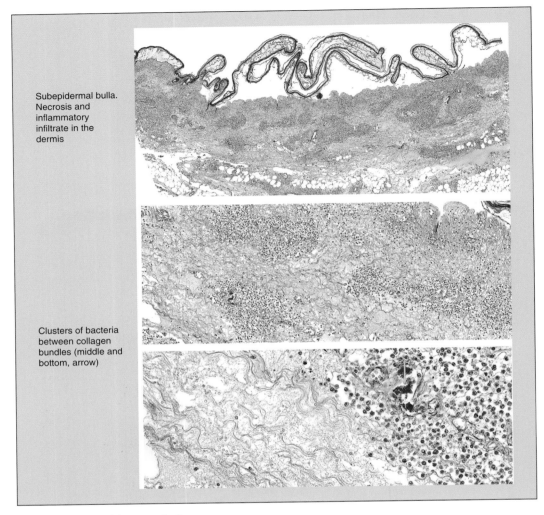

Subepidermal bulla. Necrosis and inflammatory infiltrate in the dermis

Clusters of bacteria between collagen bundles (middle and bottom, arrow)

Figure 1.1.12.2 Phlegmon, bullous.

CF: In immunodeficient patients, superficial bacterial infections (staphylococci, streptococci, and others) can rapidly spread within soft tissue, preferentially along fasciae, without respecting natural tissue compartments, and eventually evolve into necrosis of connective tissue, muscles, and fasciae.

HF:
- Epidermis partially or completely necrotic
- Subepidermal blisters and bullae
- Dermal edema, neutrophilic infiltrate, and bacteria
- Blood vessels may be thrombosed

DD: Erysipelas.

1.1.13 Necrotizing Fasciitis (Streptococcal Gangrene)°

This is a fulminant necrotizing process due to infection mostly with group A β-hemolytic streptococci. Impaired health condition and immunodeficiency are predisposing factors in this rapidly developing and often fatal disease, which may follow minor trauma or surgery.

CF: Painful erythema develops rapidly into blister formation, necrosis, and deep ulceration with subsequent gangrene.

HF:

- Blistering
- Diffuse infiltration of the dermis with neutrophils and lymphocytes
- Necrosis of soft tissue
- Involvement of fasciae and muscles
- Thrombosis with occlusion of vessels

DD: Phlegmon; panniculitis.

1.1.14 Hidradenitis Suppurativa (Acne Inversa)

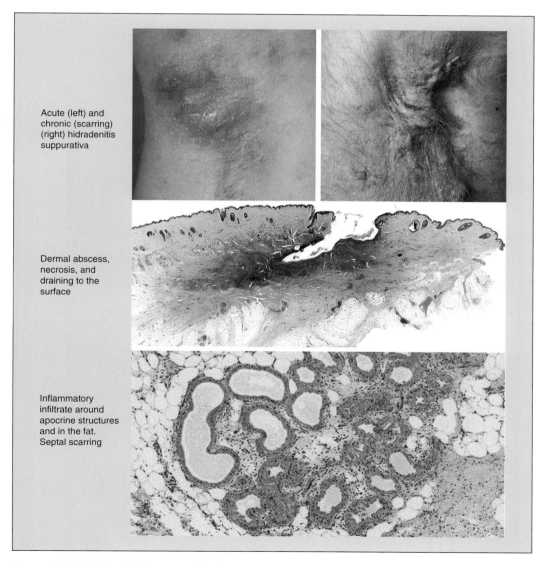

Acute (left) and chronic (scarring) (right) hidradenitis suppurativa

Dermal abscess, necrosis, and draining to the surface

Inflammatory infiltrate around apocrine structures and in the fat. Septal scarring

Figure 1.1.14 Hidradenitis Suppurativa (Acne Inversa).

CF: Areas rich in apocrine glands, such as axillae, groin, or buttocks, are preferentially involved, showing painful purulent, furunculoid nodules and scarring with sinuses and fistulas. The disease is associated with acne conglobata.

HF:

- Dermal abscesses, draining to the surface
- Mixed inflammatory infiltrate
- Neutrophils predominate
- Lymphocytes, plasma cells, eosinophils, and fibrosis in later stages
- Granulomatous reactions with multinucleated giant cells
- Scarring fibrosis and destruction of adnexal structures

DD: Granuloma inguinale; Crohn's disease; Pemphigus benignus familiaris (Hailey-Hailey); Actinomycosis; chronic fungal infection; Langerhans cell histiocytosis.

Reference

Jemec, G. B., & Hansen, U. (1996). Histology of hidradenitis suppurativa. *J Am Acad Dermatol*, **34**(6), 994–999.

Kalen, J. E., Shokeen, D., Mislankar, M., Wangia, M., & Motaparthi, K. (2018). Langerhans cell histiocytosis with clinical and histologic features of hidradenitis suppurativa: Brief report and review. *Am J Dermatopathol*, **40**(7), 502–505.

Prens, E., & Deckers, I. (2015). Pathophysiology of hidradenitis suppurativa: An update. *J Am Acad Dermatol*, **73**(5 Suppl 1), S8–11.

1.2 Other Bacterial Infections: Corynebacteria

1.2.1 Erythrasma

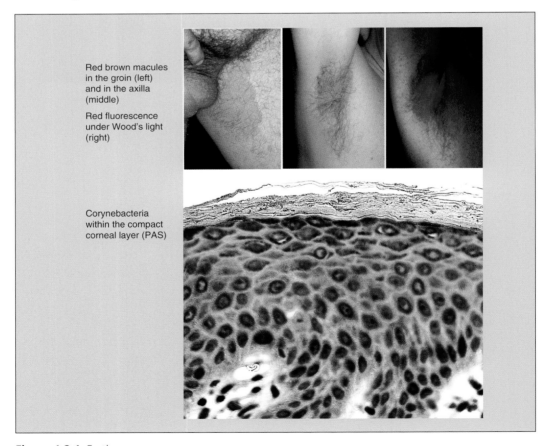

Red brown macules in the groin (left) and in the axilla (middle)

Red fluorescence under Wood's light (right)

Corynebacteria within the compact corneal layer (PAS)

Figure 1.2.1 Erythrasma.

CF: Reddish brown macules in moist intertriginous areas (groin, axillae) due to infection with bacteria *Corynebacterium minutissimum*. Coral red fluorescence under UVA light (Wood lamp).
HF:

- "Invisible" dermatosis (i.e. distinct clinical findings correlating with inconspicuous histopathological setting)

- Tiny filamentous gram-positive, PAS-positive (slightly) rods within the cornified layer
- Sparse dermal perivascular infiltrate may be present

DD: Intertrigo, trichophytia, candidiasis, toxic or allergic contact dermatitis.

1.2.2 Pitted Keratolysis (Keratoma Sulcatum)

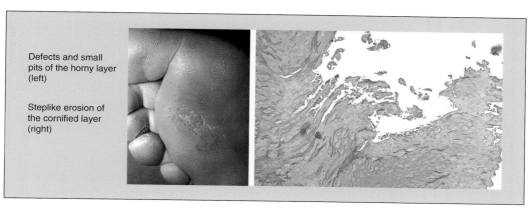

Defects and small pits of the horny layer (left)

Steplike erosion of the cornified layer (right)

Figure 1.2.2 Pitted Keratolysis (Keratoma Sulcatum).

CF: Mostly in association with hyperhidrosis (occlusive footwear), small pits are seen within the thickened macerated corneal layer of the soles, or occasionally of the palms, due to keratolytic enzymes produced by *Corynebacterium* spp. or other gram-positive bacteria.
HF: Clefts and elongated spaces within the corneal layer, containing bacteria. Missing or sparse inflammation.

Reference

de Almeida, H. L., Jr., Siqueira, R. N., Meireles Rda, S., Rampon, G., de Castro, L. A., & Silva, R. M. (2016). Pitted keratolysis. *An Bras Dermatol*, **91**(1), 106–108.

1.2.3 Trichobacteriosis (Trichomycosis) Palmellina

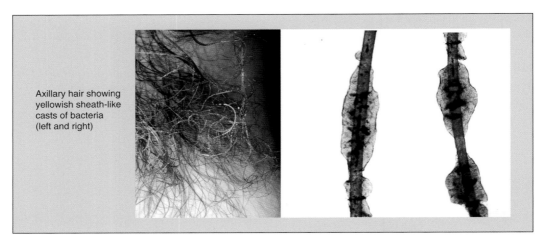

Axillary hair showing yellowish sheath-like casts of bacteria (left and right)

Figure 1.2.3 Trichobacteriosis (Trichomycosis) Palmellina.

CF: This disorder, which formerly was considered to be a fungal infection, in truth is caused by corynebacteria (*Corynebacterium tenuis*), forming white-yellow, red or black, difficult-to-remove, compact deposits along the hair shafts, preferentially in the axillae, where hyperhidrosis is a predisposing factor.

HF: The diagnosis is made clinically, or by microscopic examination of plucked hair shafts, or preferentially with Wood's lamp (UVA light), revealing red fluorescence due to bacterial protoporphyrin.

DD: Piedra; hair casts; taenia amiantacea.

Reference

Rho, N. K., & Kim, B. J. (2008). A corynebacterial triad: Prevalence of erythrasma and trichomycosis axillaris in soldiers with pitted keratolysis. *J Am Acad Dermatol*, **58**(2 Suppl), S57–58.

1.2.4 Erysipeloid

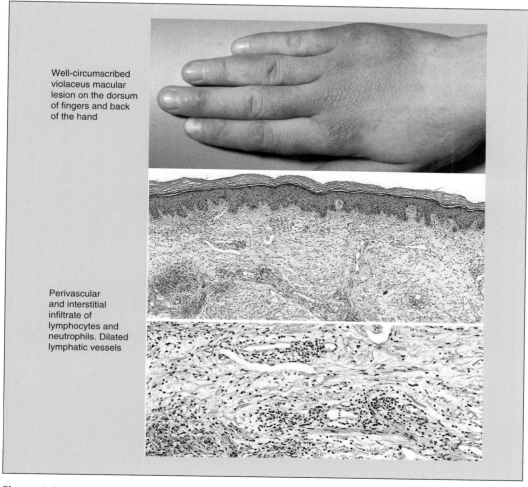

Well-circumscribed violaceus macular lesion on the dorsum of fingers and back of the hand

Perivascular and interstitial infiltrate of lymphocytes and neutrophils. Dilated lymphatic vessels

Figure 1.2.4 Erysipeloid.

This rare, acute, mostly self-limited infection, resembling erysipelas, is caused by the gram-positive bacillus *Erysipelothrix rhusiopathiae*. Infections result from direct contact with swine or contaminated animal material. Systemic symptoms, which are commonly encountered in erysipelas, as well as lymphangitis and lymphadenitis, are lacking.

CF: The painful violaceous, macular, well-circumscribed lesion usually evolves from pinpoint injuries on the hands or fingers and slowly spreads peripherally with central clearing. There may be slight diffuse swelling.

HF:

- Dermal edema
- Dilatation of lymphatic vessels
- Diffuse superficial and deep polymorphous inflammatory infiltrate showing lymphocytes, neutrophils, eosinophils, and plasma cells
- Organisms in most cases cannot be detected with histological staining
- Microbiology/molecular pathology from skin specimens reveals infectious organisms

DD: Erysipelas; erythema migrans; contact dermatitis.

Reference

Varella, T. C., & Nico, M. M. (2005). Erysipeloid. *Int J Dermatol*, **44**(6), 497–498.

1.2.5 Anthrax

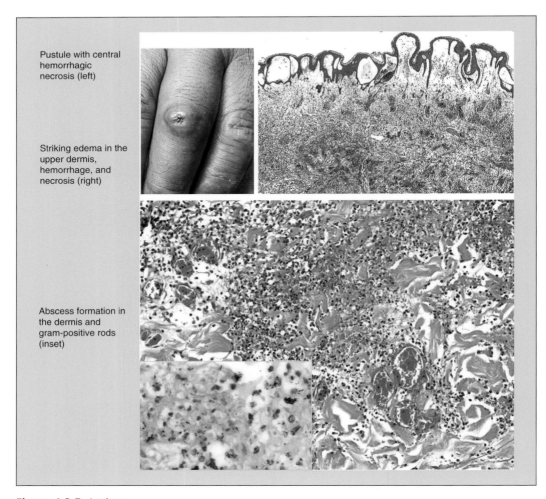

Pustule with central hemorrhagic necrosis (left)

Striking edema in the upper dermis, hemorrhage, and necrosis (right)

Abscess formation in the dermis and gram-positive rods (inset)

Figure 1.2.5 Anthrax.

The gram-positive *Bacillus anthracis* spawns permanent spores that are resistant in harsh environment, thrive in tissue, and produce exotoxins. Farmers, veterinarians, butchers, and slaughterhouse workers are especially vulnerable to infection. Remarkably, anthrax spores have been misused as biological weapons (respiratory infection).

CF: In cutaneous anthrax infection, striking edema develops at the inoculation site. A pustule forms, which becomes hemorrhagic, necrotic, and finally turns black in the center ("pustula maligna").

HF:

- Striking edema in the upper dermis
- Hemorrhage
- Necrosis
- Diffuse lymphocytic and neutrophilic infiltrate in the dermis
- Abscess formation
- Gram-positive, markedly elongated bacterial rods

DD: Sporotrichosis; orf; arthropod bite reaction; staphylococcal infection; tularemia.

Reference

Dixon, T. C., Meselson, M., Guillemin, J., & Hanna, P. C. (1999). Anthrax. *N Engl J Med*, **341**(11), 815–826.

Mallon, E., & McKee, P. H. (1997). Extraordinary case report: Cutaneous anthrax. *Am J Dermatopathol*, **19**(1), 79–82.

Tutrone, W. D., Scheinfeld, N. S., & Weinberg, J. M. (2002). Cutaneous anthrax: A concise review. *Cutis*, **69**(1), 27–33.

1.2.6 Nocardiosis

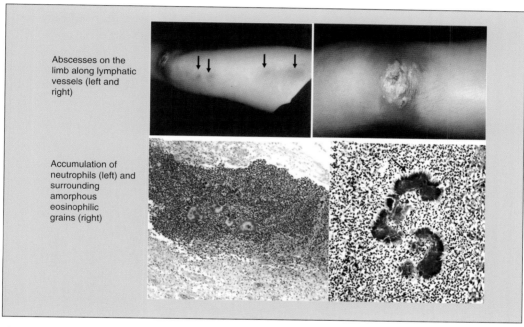

Abscesses on the limb along lymphatic vessels (left and right)

Accumulation of neutrophils (left) and surrounding amorphous eosinophilic grains (right)

Figure 1.2.6 Nocardiosis. *Source:* The images top left and right is modified from Fukuda et al. (2008). Lymphocutaneous type of nocardiosis caused by Nocardia brasiliensis: a case report and review of primary cutaneous nocardiosis caused by N. brasiliensis reported in Japan. *J Dermatol*, 35(6), 346-353. The images bottom left and right is modified from Bandeira et al. (2019). Primary cutaneous nocardiosis. *J Dtsch Dermatol Ges*. doi:10.1111/ddg.13770.

Nocardia species comprises a group of gram-positive bacteria with low or moderate virulence, which branch with filaments, and occur worldwide in soil, plants, and organic material. Cutaneous nocardiosis in most cases is caused by infection with *Nocardia brasiliensis*, mostly in immunocompromised patients.

CF: In sporotrichoid nocardiosis, abscesses develop on the limbs along lymphatic vessels.

HF:

- Suppurative infiltrate resembling actinomycosis
- Large superficial neutrophilic abscesses
- Granulomatous reaction at the periphery
- Grains with pale center, surrounded by amorphous eosinophilic (pseudoactinomycotic) bodies (Splendore–Hoeppli phenomenon)

DD: Actinomycosis; sporotrichosis; deep fungal and atypical mycobacterial infections.

Reference

Bandeira, I. D., Guimaraes-Silva, P., Cedro-Filho, R. L., de Almeida, V. R. P., Bittencourt, A. L., & Brites, C. (2019). Primary cutaneous nocardiosis. *J Dtsch Dermatol Ges*, **17**(3), 327–329.

Naka, W., Miyakawa, S., Niizeki, H., Fukuda, T., Mikami, Y., & Nishikawa, T. (1995). Unusually located lymphocutaneous nocardiosis caused by Nocardia brasiliensis. *Br J Dermatol*, **132**(4), 609–613.

Warren, N. G. (1996). Actinomycosis, nocardiosis, and actinomycetoma. *Dermatol Clin*, **14**(1), 85–95.

1.2.7 Rhinoscleroma

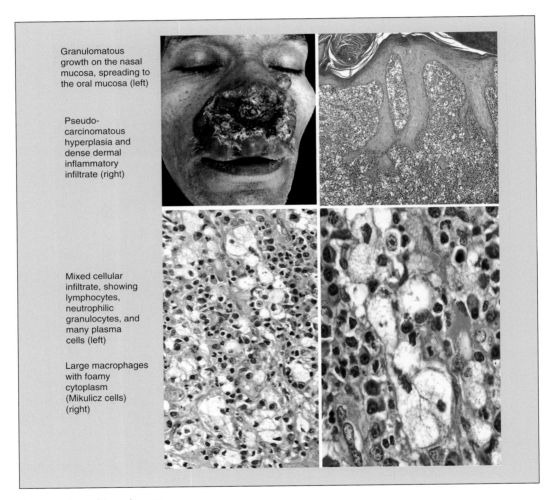

Figure 1.2.7 Rhinoscleroma.

Rare infection by the gram-negative *Klebsiella pneumoniae rhinoscleromatis*.

CF: The nasal mucosa is preferentially affected. Initially chronic rhinitis, followed by granulomatous growth on the nasal mucosa, spreading to the oral mucosa. Lesions resolve by scarring and permanent tissue destruction.

HF:

- Pseudocarcinomatous hyperplasia of the mucosa
- Mixed diffuse and dense infiltrate of the upper and lower propria
- Lymphocytes, neutrophils, and many plasma cells with Russell bodies (cytoplasmic deposits of immunoglobulin)

- Large macrophages with foamy cytoplasm and bacilli (Mikulicz cells)
- Special stains: silver, Gram, Giemsa, PAS (Russell bodies)

DD: Leishmaniasis, NK/T-cell lymphoma.

Reference

Ahmed, A. R., El-Badawy, Z. H., Mohamed, I. R., & Abdelhameed, W. A. (2015). Rhinoscleroma: A detailed histopathological diagnostic insight. *Int J Clin Exp Pathol*, **8**(7), 8438–8445.

Castanedo Cazares, J. P., & Martinez Rosales, K. I. (2015). Images in clinical medicine. Rhinoscleroma. *N Engl J Med*, **372**(25), e33.

Efared, B., Hammas, N., Gabrielle, A. E., Ben Mansour, N., El Fatemi, H., & Chbani, L. (2018). Rhinoscleroma: A chronic infectious disease of poor areas with characteristic histological features – report of a series of six cases. *Trop Doct*, **48**(1), 33–35.

1.3 Rochalimaea/Bartonellae

Gram-negative bacteria (*Bartonella henselae* or *Bartonella quintana*; formerly Rochalimaea) are the causative agent in bacillary angiomatosis, cat scratch disease, and in verruga peruana.

1.3.1 Bacillary Angiomatosis and Cat Scratch Disease

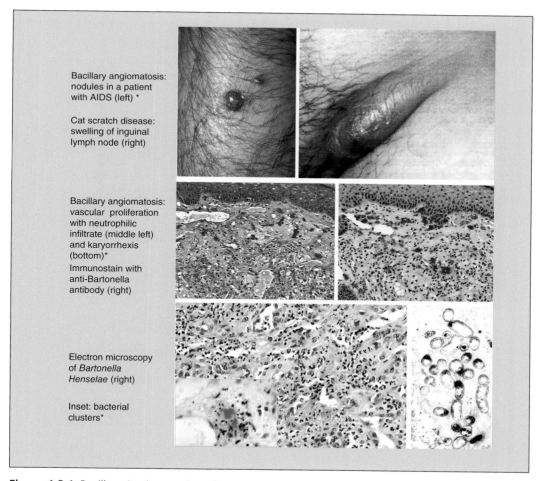

Bacillary angiomatosis: nodules in a patient with AIDS (left) *

Cat scratch disease: swelling of inguinal lymph node (right)

Bacillary angiomatosis: vascular proliferation with neutrophilic infiltrate (middle left) and karyorrhexis (bottom)*

Immunostain with anti-Bartonella antibody (right)

Electron microscopy of *Bartonella Henselae* (right)

Inset: bacterial clusters*

Figure 1.3.1 Bacillary Angiomatosis and Cat Scratch Disease (top right).
Source: Burg et al. (2019). *Atlas of Dermatopathology: Tumors, Nevi, and Cysts* (p. 273). Oxford: Wiley.

Immunodeficient patients suffering from AIDS are most commonly affected.

CF: Pyogenic granuloma-like, mostly multiple red hemorrhagic nodules or plaques. Granulomatous swelling of the draining lymph node in cat scratch disease. Concomitant internal manifestation may occur (peliosis hepatica).

HF:

- Vascular proliferation resembling pyogenic granuloma or granulation tissue
- Blood vessels with large, activated epithelioid endothelia, high mitotic activity
- Conspicuous lack of fibrous septa between capillary lobules
- Edematous stroma
- Neutrophil-rich inflammatory infiltrate with karyorrhexis
- Causative bacteria can be demonstrated by Warthin–Starry stain or immunostains, preferentially in close proximity to vessels

DD: Pyogenic granuloma (lobular capillary hemangioma); epithelioid hemangioma (angiolymphoid hyperplasia with eosinophilia); Kaposi's sarcoma; verruga peruana.

Reference

Amsbaugh, S., Huiras, E., Wang, N. S., Wever, A., & Warren, S. (2006). Bacillary angiomatosis associated with pseudoepitheliomatous hyperplasia. *Am J Dermatopathol, 28*(1), 32–35.

Kempf, V. A., Lebiedziejewski, M., Alitalo, K., Walzlein, J. H., Ehehalt, U., Fiebig, J., . . . Autenrieth, I. B. (2005). Activation of hypoxia-inducible factor-1 in bacillary angiomatosis: Evidence for a role of hypoxia-inducible factor-1 in bacterial infections. *Circulation, 111*(8), 1054–1062.

Perez-Piteira, J., Ariza, A., Mate, J. L., Ojanguren, I., & Navas-Palacios, J. J. (1995). Bacillary angiomatosis: A gross mimicker of malignancy. *Histopathology, 26*(5), 476–478.

Tsang, W. Y., Chan, J. K., & Wong, C. S. (1992). Giemsa stain for histological diagnosis of bacillary angiomatosis. *Histopathology, 21*(3): 299.

1.3.2 Verruga Peruana

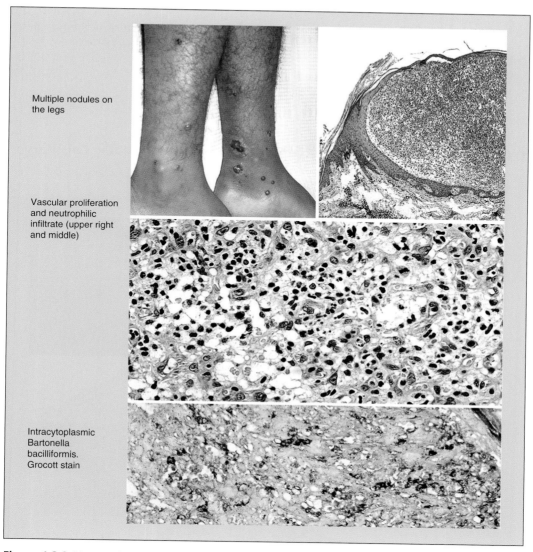

Multiple nodules on the legs

Vascular proliferation and neutrophilic infiltrate (upper right and middle)

Intracytoplasmic Bartonella bacilliformis. Grocott stain

Figure 1.3.2 Verruga Peruana.
Source: Burg et al. (2019). *Atlas of Dermatopathology: Tumors, Nevi, and Cysts* (p. 274). Oxford: Wiley.

CF: Dermal papules and nodules, pedunculated, eroded or verrucous, resembling bacillary angiomatosis. Verruga peruana is the late stage of Oroya fever that is caused by *Bartonella bacilliformis*, almost exclusively in the Andes Mountains (Peru). Infectious vectors are sandflies.

HF: Corresponds to bacillary angiomatosis, albeit with exclusively intracytoplasmic bacteria (Rocha–Lima bodies), while in bacillary angiomatosis infectious organisms thrive purely extracellularly.

DD: See bacillary angiomatosis.

Reference

Arias-Stella, J., Lieberman, P. H., Garcia-Caceres, U., Erlandson, R. A., Kruger, H., & Arias-Stella, J., Jr. (1987). Verruga peruana mimicking malignant neoplasms. *Am J Dermatopathol*, **9**(4), 279–291.

Bhutto, A. M., Nonaka, S., Hashiguchi, Y., & Gomez, E. A. (1994). Histopathological and electron microscopical features of skin lesions in a patient with bartonellosis (verruga peruana). *J Dermatol*, **21**(3), 178–184.

Jimenez-Lucho, V. (1998). Images in clinical medicine. Verruga peruana. *N Engl J Med*, **339**(7), 450.

1.3.3 Differential Diagnosis: Pyogenic Granuloma (Lobular Capillary Hemangioma; Botryomycosis)

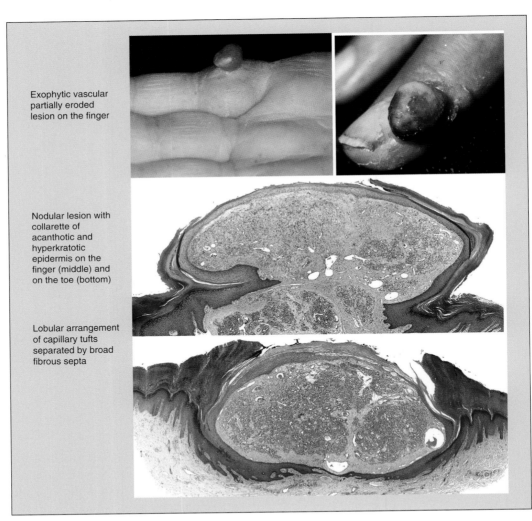

Exophytic vascular partially eroded lesion on the finger

Nodular lesion with collarette of acanthotic and hyperkratotic epidermis on the finger (middle) and on the toe (bottom)

Lobular arrangement of capillary tufts separated by broad fibrous septa

Figure 1.3.3 Differential Diagnosis: Pyogenic Granuloma (Lobular Capillary Hemangioma; Botryomycosis).
Source: Burg et al. (2019). *Atlas of Dermatopathology: Tumors, Nevi, and Cysts* (p. 270). Oxford: Wiley.

Benign vascular hyperplasia, histologically showing a lobular structure with fibrous septa and accompanied by variable inflammatory infiltrate.

CF: Soft, friable, easily vulnerable and bleeding, pedunculated exophytic nodular lesion. The lesion is surrounded by an epithelial collarette. Fingers, palms, face, and scalp are preferential sites. Pyogenic granuloma, however, may occur on any other part of the body, including oral mucosa. Superficial trauma is considered the most common cause. The growth of the lesion can be fostered by hormonal (pregnancy) and other factors (tretinoin).

HF:

- Dome-shaped lesion
- Epithelial collarette at the borders
- Flat epidermis; superficial ulceration and crust formation with bacteria are common
- Multilobular architecture with fibrous septa between vascular lobules
- Proliferation of capillaries (CD31; CD34): central "feeder vessel"
- Mitoses of endothelial cells without cellular atypia
- Variable inflammatory neutrophil-rich infiltrate and edema; predominant fibrosis in advanced lesions
- Remarkably, bacteria never occur within the center of the lesion

DD: Granulation tissue; amelanotic malignant melanoma; infantile/congenital hemangioma; nodular Kaposi sarcoma; angiosarcoma; acquired tufted angioma.

Reference

Fortna, R. R., & Junkins-Hopkins, J. M. (2007). A case of lobular capillary hemangioma (pyogenic granuloma), localized to the subcutaneous tissue, and a review of the literature. *Am J Dermatopathol*, **29**(4), 408–411.

Fukunaga, M. (2000). Kaposi's sarcoma-like pyogenic granuloma. *Histopathology*, **37**(2), 192–193.

McClain, C. M., Haws, A. L., Galfione, S. K., Rapini, R. P., & Hafeez Diwan, A. (2016). Pyogenic granuloma-like Kaposi's sarcoma. *J Cutan Pathol*, **43**(6), 549–551.

Vega Harring, S. M., Niyaz, M., Okada, S., & Kudo, M. (2004). Extramedullary hematopoiesis in a pyogenic granuloma: A case report and review. *J Cutan Pathol*, **31**(8), 555–557.

1.4 Mycobacterial Infections

Mycobacteria that cause tuberculosis and leprosy are subsumed under the heading of "typical" mycobacteria, while infections caused by *M. marinum* (swimming pool or fish tank mycobacteriosis), *M. ulcerans* (Buruli ulcer), and *M. kansasii* are commonly referred to as "atypical" mycobacterioses. Histopathologically, all mycobacteria can be detected by Ziehl–Neelsen stain (acid-fast bacilli), immunohistochemistry, or by PCR.

1.4.1 Tuberculosis Cutis

Depending on the immune status of the patient, various forms of cutaneous and subcutaneous tuberculosis of the skin occur.

Reference

Kannan, S., Simpson, G. L., Sheehan, D. J., & Lesher, J. L., Jr. (2009). Giant verrucous nodules in a patient with tuberculosis. *Am J Dermatopathol*, **31**(6), 591–593.

Maldonado-Bernal, C., Ramos-Garibay, A., Rios-Sarabia, N., Serrano, H., Carrera, M., Navarrete-Franco, G., . . . Isibasi, A. (2019). Nested Polymerase Chain Reaction and Cutaneous Tuberculosis. *Am J Dermatopathol*, **41**(6), 428–435.

Massi, D., Trotta, M., Franchi, A., Pimpinelli, N., & Santucci, M. (2004). Atypical CD30+ cutaneous lymphoid proliferation in a patient with tuberculosis infection. *Am J Dermatopathol*, **26**(3), 234–236.

Sharma, S., Sehgal, V. N., Bhattacharya, S. N., Mahajan, G., & Gupta, R. (2015). Clinicopathologic spectrum of cutaneous tuberculosis: A retrospective analysis of 165 Indians. *Am J Dermatopathol*, **37**(6), 444–450.

1.4.1.1 Primary Tuberculosis of the Skin

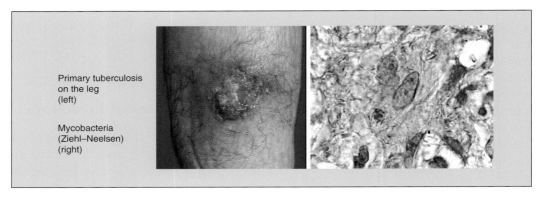

Primary tuberculosis
on the leg
(left)

Mycobacteria
(Ziehl–Neelsen)
(right)

Figure 1.4.1.1 Primary Tuberculosis of the Skin.

Primary tuberculosis of the skin, caused by *Mycobacterium tuberculosis* inoculation via superficial skin ulceration, is very rare and mostly occurs in children without previous mycobacterial contact or without Bacille Calmette-Guerin (BCG) vaccination. The immune status is anergic and the tuberculin test negative; high numbers of mycobacteria are present in the tissue.
CF: Papule or ulceration. Swelling of the draining lymph node.

HF:

- Abscess
- Necrosis
- Many mycobacteria (Ziehl–Neelsen stain)
- Granulomatous reaction occurs many weeks later

DD: Other primary mycobacterioses; foreign body granuloma; actinomycosis; sporotrichosis; tularemia.

1.4.1.2 BCG Vaccination Granuloma

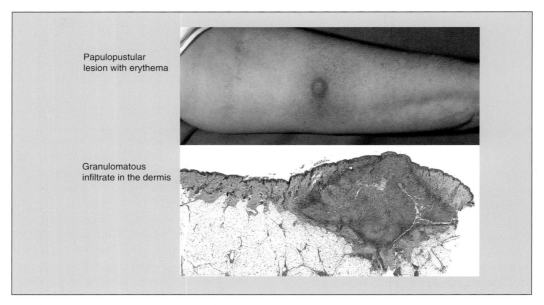

Papulopustular
lesion with erythema

Granulomatous
infiltrate in the dermis

Figure 1.4.1.2 BCG Vaccination Granuloma.

CF: Papulopustular reaction with erythema.
HF: Granulomatous inflammation with predominant epithelioid granulomas at the site of previous BCG vaccination.
DD: Insect bite; furuncle.

Reference

Keijsers, R. R., Bovenschen, H. J., & Seyger, M. M. (2011). Cutaneous complication after BCG vaccination: Case report and review of the literature. *J Dermatolog Treat*, **22**(6), 315–318.

Lyu, S. M., Choi, Y. W., Oh, C. W., Choi, H. Y., & Byun, J. Y. (2013). Granulomatous reaction after BCG vaccination histologically mimicking reticulohistiocytoma. *Eur J Dermatol*, **23**(4), 527–528.

1.4.1.3 Differential Diagnosis: Lupus Miliaris Disseminatus Faciei (LMDF)

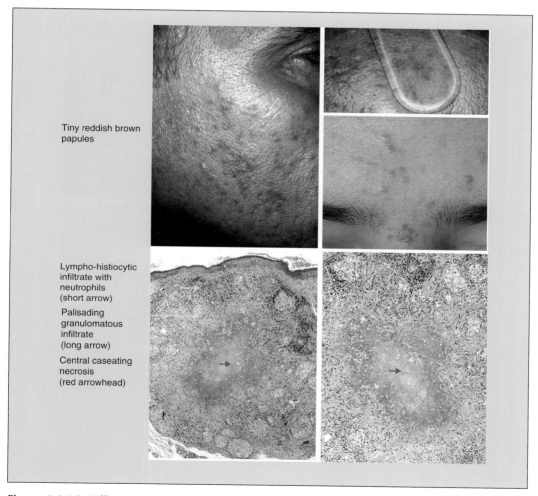

Tiny reddish brown papules

Lympho-histiocytic infiltrate with neutrophils (short arrow)

Palisading granulomatous infiltrate (long arrow)

Central caseating necrosis (red arrowhead)

Figure 1.4.1.3 Differential Diagnosis: Lupus Miliaris Disseminatus Faciei.
Source: Burg et al. (2015). *Atlas of Dermatopathology: Practical Differential Diagnosis by Clinicopathologic Pattern* (p. 184). Oxford: Wiley.

LMDF originally was considered to be a tuberculid, but eventually was subsumed under the spectrum of granulomatous rosacea or acne agminata. However, the disease occurs also in extrafacial areas.

CF: Tiny reddish brown papules, simulating acne (syn. Acne agminata and acnitis).

HF:

- Small well-circumscribed interfollicular superficial granulomas in the upper dermis
- Admixture of neutrophils
- Marked central caseating necrosis devoid of any organisms
- Peripheral wreath of densely packed histiocytes and multinucleate giant cells

- All special stains and PCR for infectious organisms are negative

DD: Acne; rosacea; verrucae planae.

Reference

Chougule, A., Chatterjee, D., Yadav, R., Sethi, S., De, D., & Saikia, U. N. (2018). Granulomatous rosacea versus lupus miliaris disseminatus faciei-2 faces of facial granulomatous disorder: A clinicohistological and molecular study. *Am J Dermatopathol*, **40**(11), 819–823.

Schaarschmidt, M. L., Schlich, M., Staub, J., Schmieder, A., Goerdt, S., & Peitsch, W. K. (2017). Lupus miliaris disseminatus faciei: Not only a facial dermatosis. *Acta Derm Venereol*, **97**(5), 655–656.

1.4.1.4 Lupus Vulgaris (LV)

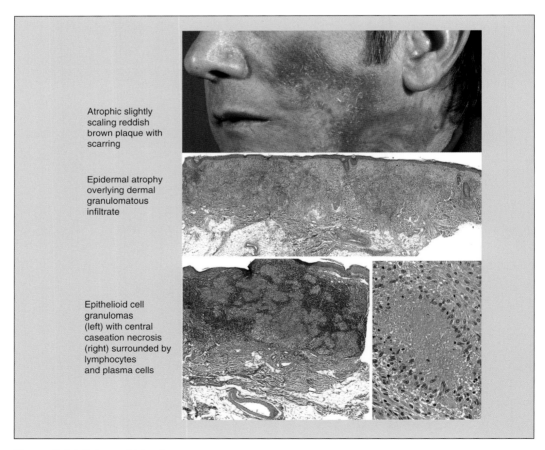

Atrophic slightly scaling reddish brown plaque with scarring

Epidermal atrophy overlying dermal granulomatous infiltrate

Epithelioid cell granulomas (left) with central caseation necrosis (right) surrounded by lymphocytes and plasma cells

Figure 1.4.1.4 Lupus Vulgaris.
Source: Burg et al. (2015). *Atlas of Dermatopathology: Practical Differential Diagnosis by Clinicopathologic Pattern* (p. 179). Oxford: Wiley.

Patients with LV have a positive Mantoux test, which indicates a normergic immune response following post-primary endogenous reactivation or secondary external inoculation.

CF: Slowly growing lesions are found mostly at acral sites, for example, ears, nose, cheeks, and peripheral parts of limbs. Tiny apple-jelly-colored reddish brown «lupoid» nodules are highly characteristic, and correlate to the granulomatous infiltrate with macrophages and multinucleate giant cells, which can be demonstrated easily by dermoscopy. Lesions resolve with atrophic and mutilating scars; recurrences are common. LV may progress to various clinical variants: verrucous, hypertrophic, ulcerating, vegetating, mutilating types of LV. Tuberculosis cutis colliquative and scrofuloderma are subcutaneous (lymph node) variants of LV.

HF:

- Epidermis is mostly atrophic, but in the verrucosus variant of LV may show pseudocarcinomatous hyperplasia

- Caseating tuberculous granulomas, composed of central necrosis, epithelioid cells, lymphocytes, multinuclear giant cells (Langhans type), plasma cells, and some neutrophils
- Fibrosis
- Infectious organisms (*M. tuberculosis*) are present in exceedingly low numbers and can almost never be detected microscopically
- Confirmation by PCR (biopsy) is difficult; conventional microbiological methods (culture) are preferred

DD: Other granulomatous infiltrates; sarcoidosis, tuberculoid leprosy; granuloma annulare; necrobiosis lipoidica; rheumatoid papule; rosacea; perioral dermatitis; deep mycosis; leishmaniasis; tertiary syphilis.

Reference

Motswaledi, M. H., & Doman, C. (2007). Lupus vulgaris with squamous cell carcinoma. *J Cutan Pathol*, **34**(12), 939–941.

1.4.1.5 Variant: Tuberculosis (Lupus) Cutis Verrucosa

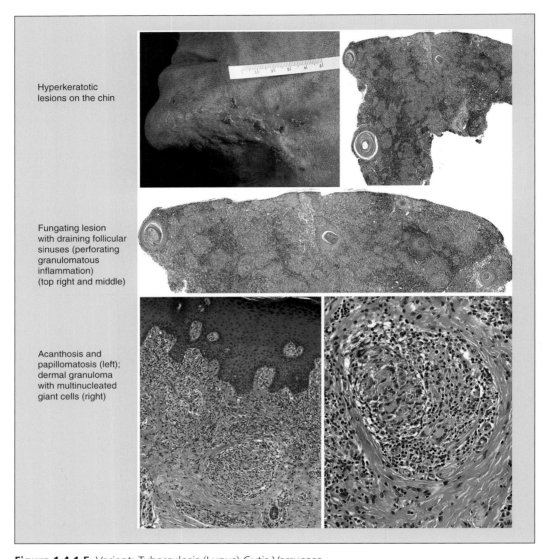

Hyperkeratotic lesions on the chin

Fungating lesion with draining follicular sinuses (perforating granulomatous inflammation) (top right and middle)

Acanthosis and papillomatosis (left); dermal granuloma with multinucleated giant cells (right)

Figure 1.4.1.5 Variant: Tuberculosis (Lupus) Cutis Verrucosa.

Variant of lupus vulgaris with overlying verrucous (pseudocarcinomatous) epidermis.

Reference

Chahar, M., Dhali, T. K., & D'Souza, P. (2015). Multifocal tuberculosis verrucosa cutis. *Dermatol Online J*, **21**(1).

Lim, J. A., Tan, W. C., Khor, B. T., Hukam Gopal Chand, S. D., & Palanivelu, T. (2017). Early onset of squamous cell carcinoma arising from tuberculosis verrucosa cutis. *J Am Coll Clin Wound Spec*, **9**(1–3), 35–38.

1.4.1.6 Variant: Tuberculosis Cutis Colliquativa (Scrofuloderma)

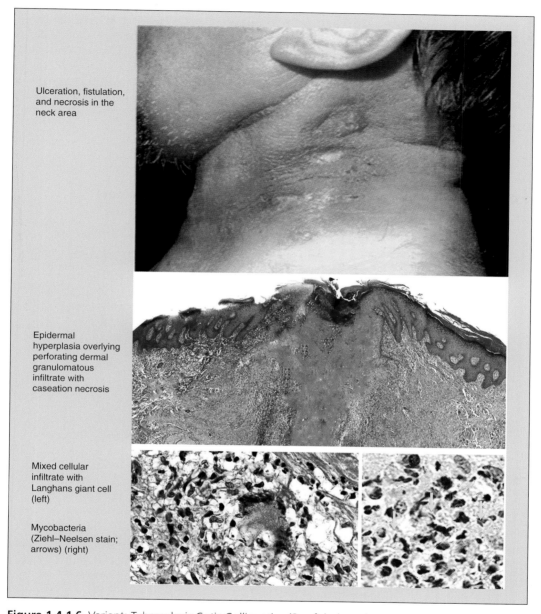

Ulceration, fistulation, and necrosis in the neck area

Epidermal hyperplasia overlying perforating dermal granulomatous infiltrate with caseation necrosis

Mixed cellular infiltrate with Langhans giant cell (left)

Mycobacteria (Ziehl–Neelsen stain; arrows) (right)

Figure 1.4.1.6 Variant: Tuberculosis Cutis Colliquativa (Scrofuloderma).

Chronic subcutaneous variant of tuberculosis with underlying normergic immune status.

CF: Skin involvement may result from per continuitatem draining infected lymph nodes in the head and neck area. Typical are painless swelling and ulceration with necrosis and fistulation, leading to adherence of the overlying skin and finally scar formation.

HF:

- Nonspecific epidermal hyperplasia
- Massive necrosis
- Tuberculoid granulomas with Langhans giant cells
- Mixed inflammatory infiltrate with lymphocytes, plasma cells, and neutrophils
- Tuberculous pus

DD: Actinomycosis; deep fungal infections; lymphogranuloma; tertiary syphilis (gumma).

Reference

Gupta, M., Gupta, M., & Kaur, R. (2013). Tuberculosis colliquativa cutis of the cheek: An extremely uncommon manifestation of primary extrapulmonary tuberculosis. *BMJ Case Rep, 2013.*

Tur, E., Brenner, S., & Meiron, Y. (1996). Scrofuloderma (tuberculosis colliquativa cutis). *Br J Dermatol*, **134**(2), 350–352.

1.4.1.7 Lichen Scrofulosorum (Tuberculosis Cutis Lichenoides)

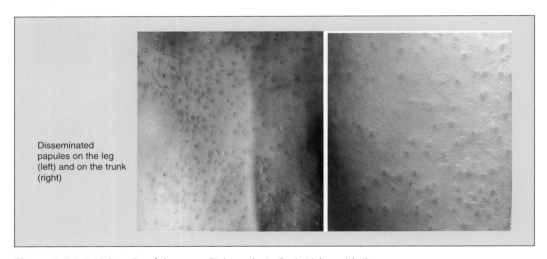

Disseminated papules on the leg (left) and on the trunk (right)

Figure 1.4.1.7 Lichen Scrofulosorum (Tuberculosis Cutis Lichenoides).

Hyperergic immune status, showing strongly positive tuberculin test. *Mycobacteria* usually cannot be detected in the tissue, although they may be present in very low numbers.

CF: Tiny reddish brown follicular or perifollicular papules clustered ("lichenoid") in a circumscribed area of the trunk or extremities. Remarkable morphological overlap with lichen nitidus.

HF:

- Follicular or perifollicular granulomatous infiltrate
- Epithelioid cell infiltrate with some Langhans giant cells
- Lymphocytes and histiocytes between tuberculoid nodules
- Rarely, mycobacteria may be detectable in some cases by special stains (Ziehl–Neelsen) or by PCR

DD: Lichen (ruber) planus; lichen nitidus; lichen syphiliticus; lichen trichophyticus

Reference

Ben Jazia, E., Hachfi, W., Trimech, M., Hmissa, S., Jeddi, C. H., & Omezzine-Letaief, A. (2006). Detection of mycobacterial tuberculosis DNA in lichen scrofulosorum. *J Am Acad Dermatol*, **55**(2 Suppl), S54–55.

Camacho, D., Pielasinski, U., Revelles, J. M., Gorgolas, M., Manzarbeitia, F., Kutzner, H., & Requena, L. (2011). Lichen scrofulosorum mimicking lichen planus. *Am J Dermatopathol*, **33**(2), 186–191.

1.4.1.8 Papulonecrotic Tuberculid

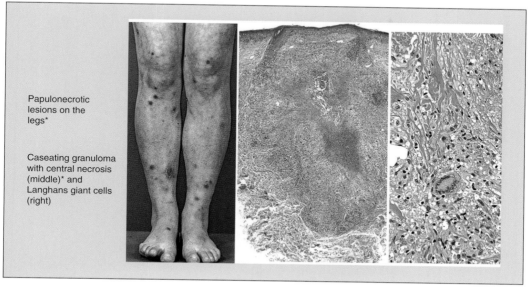

Papulonecrotic lesions on the legs*

Caseating granuloma with central necrosis (middle)* and Langhans giant cells (right)

Figure 1.4.1.8 Papulonecrotic Tuberculid.
*Source: Burg et al. (2015). *Atlas of Dermatopathology. Practical Differential Diagnosis by Clinicopathologic Pattern* (p. 182). Oxford: Wiley.

Immune status as in lichen scrofulosorum, that is, hyperergic with strongly positive tuberculin test.

CF: Symmetric disseminated erythematous papulonecrotic and ulcerated lesions, mostly in acral localization; resolving with scar formation.

HF:

- Wedge-shaped infiltrate in the dermis
- Granulomatous infiltrate with caseous necrosis
- Giant multinuclear cells (Langhans giant cells)
- Concomitant lymphocytic vasculitis
- Thrombosed blood vessels
- Mycobacteria completely lacking (negative Ziehl–Neelsen stain)

- PCR/culture for mycobacteria may be positive

DD: Pityriasis lichenoides et varioliformis acuta (PLEVA); leukocytoclastic vasculitis; prurigo.

Reference

Jordaan, H. F., Van Niekerk, D. J., & Louw, M. (1994). Papulonecrotic tuberculid. A clinical, histopathological, and immunohistochemical study of 15 patients. *Am J Dermatopathol*, **16**(5), 474–485.

Victor, T., Jordaan, H. F., Van Niekerk, D. J., Louw, M., Jordaan, A., & Van Helden, P. D. (1992). Papulonecrotic tuberculid. Identification of Mycobacterium tuberculosis DNA by polymerase chain reaction. *Am J Dermatopathol*, **14**(6), 491–495.

1.4.1.9 Erythema Induratum Bazin

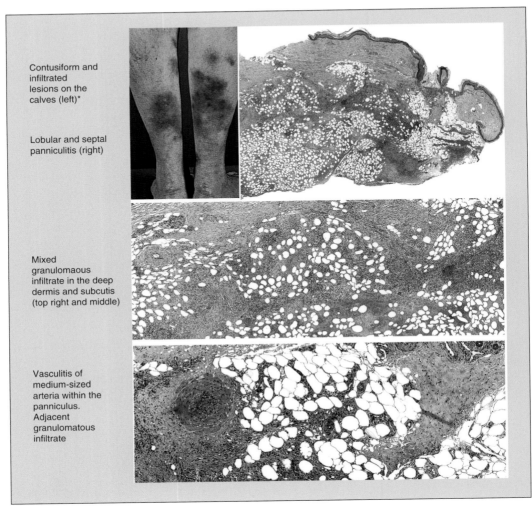

Contusiform and infiltrated lesions on the calves (left)*

Lobular and septal panniculitis (right)

Mixed granulomaous infiltrate in the deep dermis and subcutis (top right and middle)

Vasculitis of medium-sized arteria within the panniculus. Adjacent granulomatous infiltrate

Figure 1.4.1.9 Erythema Induratum (Bazin).
*Source: Burg et al. (2015). *Atlas of Dermatopathology: Practical Differential Diagnosis by Clinicopathologic Pattern* (p. 183). Oxford: Wiley.

"Classic" EIB is a subcutaneous variant of hyperergic reaction in patients who have or have had tuberculosis. The tuberculin test is strongly positive. Non-tuberculous variants of EIB may occur, clinically and histopathologically often overlapping with nodular vasculitis.

CF: Contusiform plaques and intradermal nodular infiltration, often located on the calves, simulating vasculitis or thrombophlebitis. Ulceration is rare, but may occur at advanced stages.

HF:
- Lobular panniculitis, occasionally evolving into suppurative panniculitis
- Granulomatous perivascular infiltrates, mostly in the deep dermal plexus
- Lipophagic granulomas in advanced lesions

- Nodular arterial subcutaneous vasculitis is not an inherent part of "classic" EIB

DD: Nodular vasculitis, erythema nodosum; sarcoidosis; pernio

Reference

Roblin, D., Kelly, R., Wansbrough-Jones, M., & Harwood, C. (1994). Papulonecrotic tuberculide and erythema induratum as presenting manifestations of tuberculosis. *J Infect*, **28**(2), 193–197.

Wang, T. C., Tzen, C. Y., & Su, H. Y. (2000). Erythema induratum associated with tuberculous lymphadenitis: Analysis of a case using polymerase chain reactions with different primer pairs to differentiate bacille Calmette-Guerin (BCG) from virulent strains of Mycobacterium tuberculosis complex. *J Dermatol*, **27**(11), 717–723.

1.4.2 Atypical Mycobacteriosis: Fish Tank (Swimming Pool) Granuloma

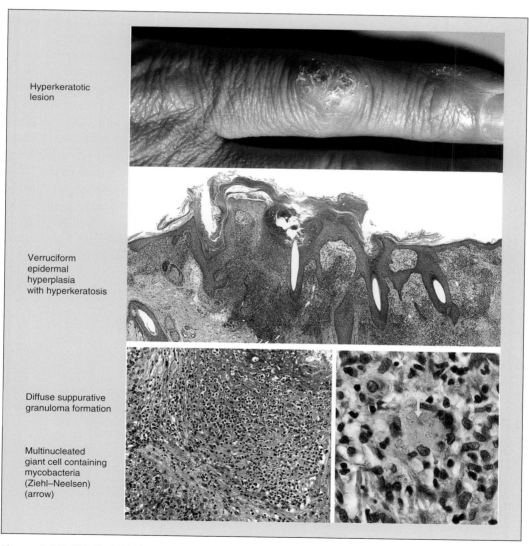

Hyperkeratotic lesion

Verruciform epidermal hyperplasia with hyperkeratosis

Diffuse suppurative granuloma formation

Multinucleated giant cell containing mycobacteria (Ziehl–Neelsen) (arrow)

Figure 1.4.2 Fish Tank (Swimming Pool) Granuloma.

Inoculation with *Mycobacterium marinum* occurs via local trauma and exposure to infested water, mostly in fish tanks or swimming pools.

CF: Hyperkeratotic lichenoid and granulomatous lesion with superficial ulceration and crust formation.

HF:

- Acanthosis and hyperkeratosis of overlying epidermis
- Tuberculoid granulomas
  - Central necrosis often present
  - Macrophages and multinucleated Langhans giant cells
  - Mixed adjacent inflammatory infiltrate, with neutrophils and lymphocytes
  - Ziehl–Neelsen stain often positive showing few microorganisms
- Fibrosis

DD: Other chronic infections and diseases associated with granulomas and mixed inflammatory dermal infiltrates.

Reference

Boyd, A. S., & Robbins, J. (2005). Cutaneous Mycobacterium avium intracellulare infection in an HIV+ patient mimicking histoid leprosy. *Am J Dermatopathol*, **27**(1), 39–41.

Breza T, J., & Magro, C. M. (2006). Lichenoid and granulomatous dermatitis associated with atypical mycobacterium infections. *J Cutan Pathol*, **33**(7), 512–515.

Redbord, K. P., Shearer, D. A., Gloster, H., Younger, B., Connelly, B. L., Kindel, S. E., & Lucky, A. W. (2006). Atypical Mycobacterium furunculosis occurring after pedicures. *J Am Acad Dermatol*, **54**(3), 520–524.

1.4.3 Leprosy (Hansen Disease)[1]

Leprosy is caused by the acid-fast *Mycobacterium leprae*, which was identified by the Norwegian physician Gerhard Armauer Hansen (1874). The armadillo is a natural carrier and serves as a vector, without becoming ill. Culturing of M. leprae has not been successful.

Lepra predominantly affects the skin and preferentially the sensory nerves (pain and temperature) and is still considered a serious health concern in many tropical and subtropical countries. The incubation period is very long (3–5 years). The Ridley–Jopling (R-J) classification of leprosy is widely used.

The early stage is called "indeterminate lepra" and shows hypopigmented (dark-skinned people) or slightly red (fair skin) spots. Histologically there may be minimal inflammation with a few bacteria present. Depending on the patient's immune status, tuberculoid, borderline, lepromatous lepra and intermediate forms may evolve. For monitoring therapy, the bacterial index (1–6; depending on the number of bacteria found in the skin) and the morphologic index (percentage of solid staining bacteria) are applied. For the demonstration of lepra bacilli in the tissue, the Fite-Faraco stain is more suitable than the Ziehl–Neelsen method. In situ hybridization and PCR analysis of specimens are more sensitive.

Reference

Jerath, V. P., & Desai, S. R. (1998). Diversities in clinical and histopathological classification of leprosy. *Lepr India*, **54**, 130–134.

Walkar, S. L., & Lockwood, D. N. (2006). The clinical and immunological features of leprosy. *Br Med Bull*, **78**, 174–176.

---

[1] This chapter was prepared in cooperation with Ram Chandra Adhikari MD, Consultant Dermatopathologist, DISHARC Hospital, Kathmandu/Nepal

1.4.3.1 Tuberculoid Leprosy

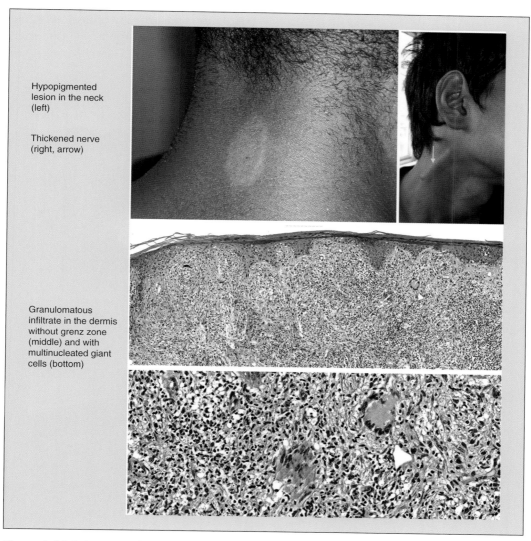

Hypopigmented lesion in the neck (left)

Thickened nerve (right, arrow)

Granulomatous infiltrate in the dermis without grenz zone (middle) and with multinucleated giant cells (bottom)

Figure 1.4.3.1 Leprosy, Tuberculoid (Paucibacillary) (TT).

Tuberculoid leprosy is seen in individuals with intact cell-mediated immunity and is associated with high resistance to the lepra bacilli. The lepromin test is strongly positive.

CF: Preferentially on the trunk and limbs there are single or few asymmetrically distributed anesthetic, anhidrotic macules or plaques with a sharply defined border. The skin is dry, scaly, erythematous, or hypopigmented. One or two nerves near the skin lesion may be thickened. Internal organs are not involved. Loss of pain and sensory functions may lead to injuries and mutilations on the acra.

HF:

- Epithelioid granulomas with Langhans multinucleated giant cells and many lymphocytes, a few plasma cells, and eosinophils

- Infiltrates sometimes along nerves
- No grenz zone
- No caseous necrosis
- Partly destroyed dermal nerves by granulomas are diagnostic for leprosy

- Granulomas may erode the epidermis
- Acid-fast bacilli are rare or absent

DD: Lupus vulgaris; sarcoidosis; leishmaniasis; xanthomas; granular cell tumor.

1.4.3.2 Borderline Leprosy

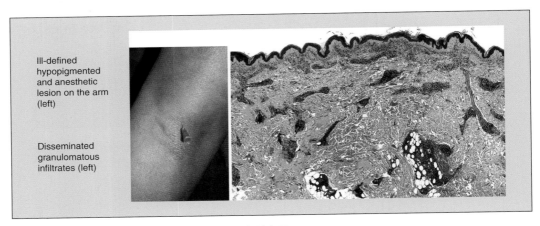

Ill-defined hypopigmented and anesthetic lesion on the arm (left)

Disseminated granulomatous infiltrates (left)

Figure 1.4.3.2.1 Leprosy: Borderline Tuberculoid (BT).

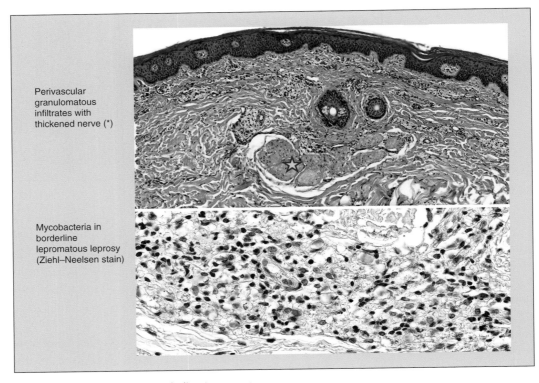

Perivascular granulomatous infiltrates with thickened nerve (*)

Mycobacteria in borderline lepromatous leprosy (Ziehl–Neelsen stain)

Figure 1.4.3.2.2 Leprosy, Borderline Lepromatous.

Borderline leprosy is an unstable form, constituting 10–15% of cases of leprosy and can progress to either pole (tuberculoid or lepromatous), depending on the immune status. The lepromin test is positive or negative.

CF: Variable lesions between lepromatous and tuberculoid leprosy. Multiple erythematous copper-colored patches of various size and shape with punched-out center and ill-defined border are seen. These lesions tend to be symmetrical. Nerves may be irregularly thickened.

HF:

- Ill-defined granulomas with unbalanced mixture of epithelioid cells, lymphocytes, and macrophages
- Langhans multinucleated giant cells are usually absent
- Mycobacteria may be present, especially in the BL-variant

DD: Lupus vulgaris; Leishmaniasis.

1.4.3.3 Lepromatous Leprosy

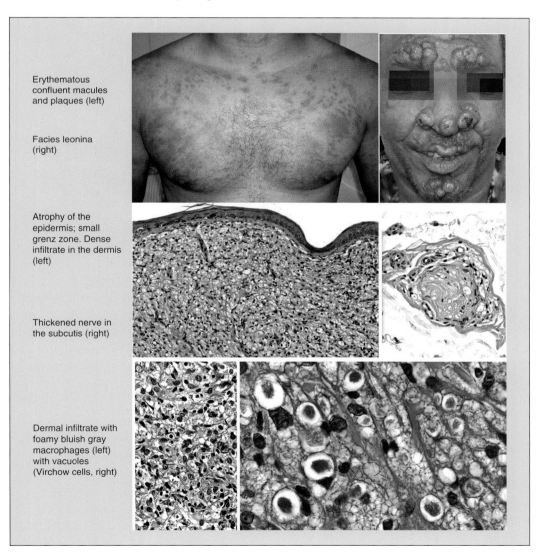

Erythematous confluent macules and plaques (left)

Facies leonina (right)

Atrophy of the epidermis; small grenz zone. Dense infiltrate in the dermis (left)

Thickened nerve in the subcutis (right)

Dermal infiltrate with foamy bluish gray macrophages (left) with vacuoles (Virchow cells, right)

Figure 1.4.3.3 Leprosy, Lepromatous (LL).

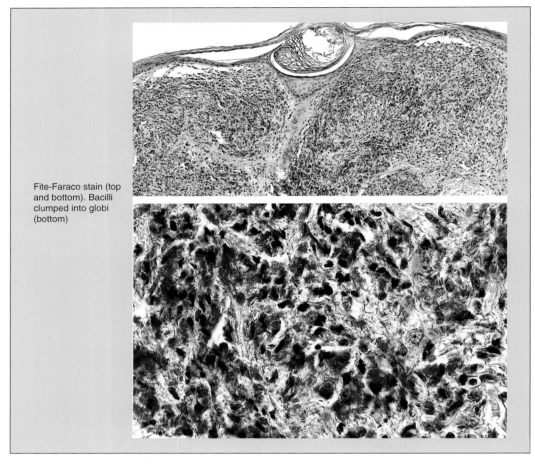

Fite-Faraco stain (top and bottom). Bacilli clumped into globi (bottom)

Figure 1.4.3.3 (Continued)

Lepromatous leprosy occurs in individuals with poor cell-mediated immunity to *M. leprae*. The lepromin test is negative. Sensation may be intact.

CF: Numerous hypopigmented or erythematous partly confluent macules, plaques, nodules, or diffusely infiltrating lesions (leonine facies) occur. They are symmetrically distributed on the face, trunk, and extremities and show ill-defined borders. Nerves are symmetrically enlarged. Internal organs may become involved.

HF:

- Thin atrophic epidermis with grenz zone
- Dermis shows numerous foamy bluish-gray macrophages with vacuoles, loaded with *M. leprae* (Virchow cells), diffusely arranged or in large sheets, replacing skin adnexal structures
- Lymphocytes are very few in number; however, there may be perineural and intraneural infiltration of nerves by lymphocytes
- Numerous M. leprae are seen with Fite-Faraco stain

DD: Atypical mycobacterial infections; xanthoma; molluscum contagiosum.

Reference

Santos-Arroyo, A. E., Nevares-Pomales, O. W., Almodovar, P. I., & Sanchez, J. L. (2014). Molluscum-like lesions in a 12-year-old boy: Challenge. Lepromatous leprosy. *Am J Dermatopathol*, **36**(12), 984, 992.

1.4.3.4 Variant: Histoid Lepromatous

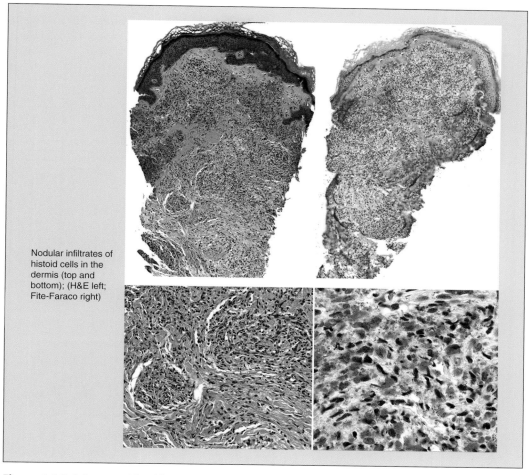

Nodular infiltrates of histoid cells in the dermis (top and bottom); (H&E left; Fite-Faraco right)

Figure 1.4.3.4 Leprosy, Histoid Lepromatous (HL).

This is an uncommon variant of lepromatous leprosy occurring in patients with lepromatous leprosy and inadequate or irregular therapy.

CF: Single or multiple well demarcated dermatofibroma-like cutaneous and subcutaneous deep-seating nodules arising on normal skin.

HF:

- Atrophy of the epidermis
- Subepidermal grenz zone
- Interlacing bundles of spindle-shaped fusiform histiocytes in the dermis arranged in storiform or crisscross pattern

- High bacillary index, without globi formation of lepra bacilli
- Histologic variants comprise pure fusocellular, fusocellular with epithelioid component, and fusocellular with vacuolated (foamy) cells

DD: Fibrous histiocytoma (dermatofibroma); keloid; erythema nodosum leprosum; sarcoidosis; reticulohistiocytosis; cutaneous metastases; atypical mycobacteriosis; molluscum.

Reference

Kalla, G., Purohit, S., & Vyas, M. C. (2000). Histoid, a clinical variant of multibacillary leprosy: Report from so-called nonendemic areas. *Int J Lepr Other Mycobact Dis,* **68**(3), 267–271.

Punia, R. P. S., Dhingra, H., Baliyan, A., Handa, U., Mohan, H., & Thami, G. P. (2017). Clinicopathologic spectrum of histoid lepra *International Journal of Current Research,* **9**(5), 50765–50769.

Rodrigues Daxbacher, E. L., Cabrera Pereira, J. P., Ramos de Oliveira, S., Duarte Tortelly, V., Carneiro, S., & Jeunon, T. (2020). The importance of the biopsy technique in the diagnosis of histoid leprosy. *Am J Dermatopathol,* **42**(2),125–128.

1.4.3.5 Variant: Erythema Nodosum Leprosum

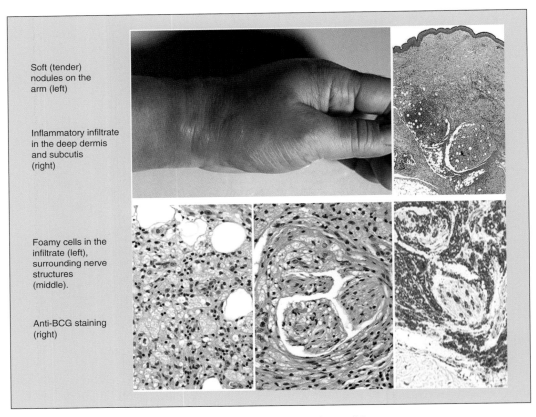

Soft (tender) nodules on the arm (left)

Inflammatory infiltrate in the deep dermis and subcutis (right)

Foamy cells in the infiltrate (left), surrounding nerve structures (middle).

Anti-BCG staining (right)

Figure 1.4.3.5 Virchow cell-rich variant of ENL with minimal vasculitis.

Various immunological reactions may be seen in conjunction with (lepromatous) leprosy. A shift toward the tuberculoid pole with better immune status under treatment is referred to as type 1 (lepra) reaction. The Lucio phenomenon, presenting as small vessel vasculitis with hemorrhagic plaques (erythema necroticans), is called type 3 reaction and is seen in patients with diffuse lepromatous leprosy. Erythema nodosum leprosum, referred to as a type 2 inflammatory reaction, shows a shift of the immune status toward the lepromatous pole with a high bacterial index. **CF**: Erythema nodosum leprosum (type 2 reaction) presents as multiple, tender, contusiform red or violaceous swelling and nodules, preferentially on the extremities. Bullous variants have been reported. **HF**: ENL is an immune complex-mediated necrotizing vasculitis involving capillaries, arterioles, arteries, venules, and veins.

- Dermis and subcutaneous tissue are involved
- Small vessel vasculitis with endothelial swelling and fibrinoid necrosis
- Fibrin in vessel walls
- Focal necrosis
- Perivascular lymphocytic and neutrophilic infiltrates and nuclear debris
- Foamy macrophages containing numerous bacilli

DD: Other forms of nodular erythema.

Reference

Bakshi, N., Rao, S., & Batra, R. (2017). Bullous erythema nodosum leprosum as the first manifestation of multibacillary leprosy: A rare phenomenon. *Am J Dermatopathol*, **39**(11), 857–859.

Kutzner, H., Argenyi, Z. B., Requena, L., Rutten, A., & Hugel, H. (1998). A new application of BCG antibody for rapid screening of various tissue microorganisms. *J Am Acad Dermatol*, **38**(1), 56–60.

1.4.4 Buruli Ulcer

CF: Even minor injury may be followed by infection with *Mycobacterium ulcerans*. Characteristically infections occur in tropical areas (Australia, Africa: Buruli is a district of Uganda) and slowly evolve into papules or nodules followed by painless ulceration with subsequent mutilation of local tissue.

HF:

- Marked necrosis with complete destruction of local tissue
- Very sparse inflammation, starting in the septal portion of the subcutaneous fat
- Giant cells
- Organisms at the borders of the ulcer (Ziehl–Neelsen)

DD: Ecthyma; squamous cell carcinoma; melanoma.

Reference

Portaels, F., Silva, M. T., & Meyers, W. M. (2009). Buruli ulcer. *Clin Dermatol*, **27**(3), 291–305.

Walsh, D. S., Portaels, F., & Meyers, W. M. (2008). Buruli ulcer (Mycobacterium ulcerans infection). *Trans R Soc Trop Med Hyg*, **102**(10), 969–978.

Zavattaro, E., Boccafoschi, F., Borgogna, C., Conca, A., Johnson, R. C., Sopoh, G. E., . . . Valente, G. (2012). Apoptosis in Buruli ulcer: A clinicopathological study of 45 cases. *Histopathology*, **61**(2), 224–236.

1.5 **Actinomycosis**

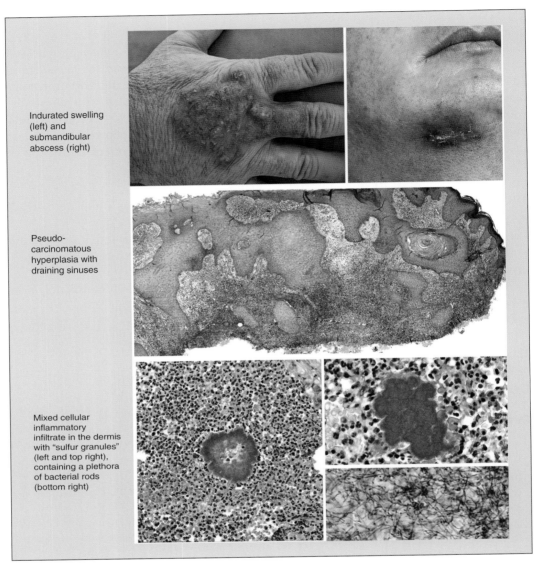

Indurated swelling (left) and submandibular abscess (right)

Pseudo-carcinomatous hyperplasia with draining sinuses

Mixed cellular inflammatory infiltrate in the dermis with "sulfur granules" (left and top right), containing a plethora of bacterial rods (bottom right)

Figure 1.5 Actinomycosis.

The anaerobic saprophytic gram-positive bacterium *Actinomyces israelii* thrives in the autochthonous flora of the mouth and the gastrointestinal tract of healthy individuals. *Actinomyces israelii* is also the most common cause of chronic suppurative infection of the mucosa, often in the course of dental or surgical procedures.

Pulmonary or gastrointestinal involvement is not unusual.

CF: Typical clinical features are erythema and concomitant indurated swelling, subsequent abscess formation, and purulent discharge with tiny granules draining through sinusoidal tracts into the cervicofacial premandibular area.

HF:

- Pseudocarcinomatous mucosal hyperplasia
- Purulent suppurative infiltrate
- Neutrophils, eosinophils, plasma cells, histiocytes
- Basophilic aggregates of *Actinomyces* organisms ("sulfur granules")
- *Actinomyces* can be detected by Giemsa or Gomori silver stains
  - in smears
  - in histological specimens
  - by cultivation
- Fibrotic induration and scarring

DD: Scrofuloderma, gumma (tertiary syphilis), lymphogranuloma venereum, Nocardiosis, metastases

Reference

Cirillo-Hyland, V., Herzberg, A., & Jaworsky, C. (1993). Cervicofacial actinomycosis resembling a ruptured cyst. *J Am Acad Dermatol*, **29**(2 Pt 2), 308–311.

De, D., Dogra, S., Kanwar, A. J., & Saikia, U. N. (2011). Actinomycosis presenting as a destructive ulcerated plaque on the palate and gingiva. *J Am Acad Dermatol*, **65**(6), 1235–1236.

1.6 Borrelia Infections (Lyme Disease)

Lyme disease, named after a small town in Connecticut, is caused by the spirochete *Borrelia burgdorferi*, transmitted by the tick Ixodes dammini (North America) or Ixodes ricinus (Europe).

Early (stage I) disease presents with a slowly expanding erythema (chronicum) migrans. If not treated, systemic neurologic, cardiac, and other symptoms as well as additional skin lesions may develop (stage II) due to hematogenous spread of the bacteria. In late disease (stage III), edema eventually transforms into atrophic (wrinkled "cigarette paper-like") skin (acrodermatitis chronica atrophicans), which may be accompanied by juxta-articular fibroid nodules and migratory monarthritis.

Serologic tests (specific IgM antibodies) and/or detection of Borrelia sp. DNA by PCR confirm the diagnosis.

Reference

Kempf, W., Kazakov, D. V., Hubscher, E., Gugerli, O., Gerbig, A. W., Schmid, R., . . . Kutzner, H. (2015). Cutaneous borreliosis associated with T cell-predominant infiltrates: A diagnostic challenge. *J Am Acad Dermatol*, **72**(4), 683–689.

Kempf, W., Kazakov, D. V., Hubscher, E., & Tinguely, M. (2015). Cutaneous borreliosis with a T-cell-rich infiltrate and simultaneous involvement by B-cell chronic lymphocytic leukemia with t(14,18)(q32;q21). *Am J Dermatopathol*, **37**(9), 715–718.

1.6.1 Variant: Erythema (Chronicum) Migrans (ECM) (Stage I)

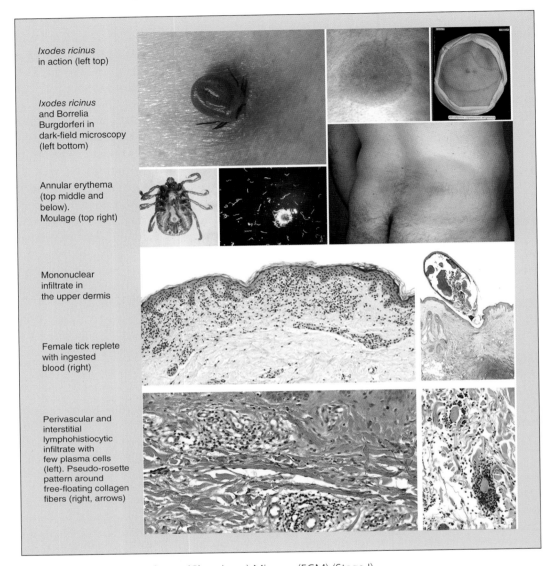

Ixodes ricinus in action (left top)

Ixodes ricinus and Borrelia Burgdorferi in dark-field microscopy (left bottom)

Annular erythema (top middle and below). Moulage (top right)

Mononuclear infiltrate in the upper dermis

Female tick replete with ingested blood (right)

Perivascular and interstitial lymphohistiocytic infiltrate with few plasma cells (left). Pseudo-rosette pattern around free-floating collagen fibers (right, arrows)

Figure 1.6.1 Variant: Erythema (Chronicum) Migrans (ECM) (Stage I).

CF: ECM, which is typically an erythematous, slowly expanding annular patch, appears at the site of a previous tick bite. A few weeks later, after the erythema has faded, a papule or a small nodule (lymphadenosis cutis benigna, lymphocytoma cutis: see below) may develop at the site of the tick bite or at a distant site, following hematogenous spread of the spirochetes (stage II).

HF: The diagnosis is based on the patient's history, clinical presentation, and serologic tests/PCR, respectively. Immunohistochemical demonstration of spirochetes is rarely feasible. In the center of the lesion, chitinous remnants of the tick (hypostome) and a neutrophil-rich inflammatory infiltrate followed by granulomatous changes may occur.

- Erythematous patch or peripheral annular rims
  - Missing or only slight spongiosis with exocytosis
  - Sparse patchy lymphoplasmacytic perivascular or interstitial (Indian file-like) infiltrate in the upper dermis
  - Eosinophils in early stages more frequent
  - Interstitial lymphohistiocytic infiltrate, sometimes in pseudo-rosette pattern around free-floating collagen fibers
    - Plasma cells, with diffuse splaying in the upper dermis, may be rare
- Center of the lesion
  - Eczematous changes of the epidermis
  - Chitinous remnants of the tick (hypostome)
  - Slight edema with dilated blood vessels
  - Mixed inflammatory cell infiltrate
  - Eosinophils (early stages) and plasma cells (advanced stages) commonly occur
  - Granulomatous reaction (advanced lesions)
  - Spirochetes can be identified only in exceptional cases (immunohistochemistry)

DD: Erysipelas; insect bite; acute urticaria (hives); tinea; all other annular (allergic) erythemas.

Reference

Celebi Cherukuri, N., Roth, C. G., Aggarwal, N., Ho, J., Gehris, R., & Akilov, O. E. (2016). Cutaneous small/medium CD4+ pleomorphic T-cell lymphoma-like nodule in a patient with erythema chronicum migrans. *Am J Dermatopathol*, **38**(6), 448–452.

Wilson, T. C., Legler, A., Madison, K. C., Fairley, J. A., & Swick, B. L. (2012). Erythema migrans: A spectrum of histopathologic changes. *Am J Dermatopathol*, **34**(8), 834–837.

1.6.2 Variant: Lymphadenosis Cutis Benigna (Pseudolymphoma, Lymphocytoma Cutis) (Stage I)

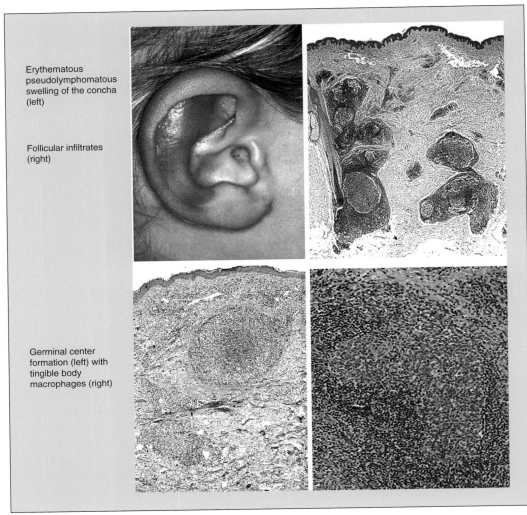

Erythematous pseudolymphomatous swelling of the concha (left)

Follicular infiltrates (right)

Germinal center formation (left) with tingible body macrophages (right)

Figure 1.6.2.1 Variant: Lymphadenosis Cutis Benigna (Pseudolymphoma; Lymphocytoma Cutis) (Stage I).
Source: Burg et al. (2019). *Atlas of Dermatopathology: Tumors, Nevi, and Cysts* (p. 393). Oxford: Wiley.

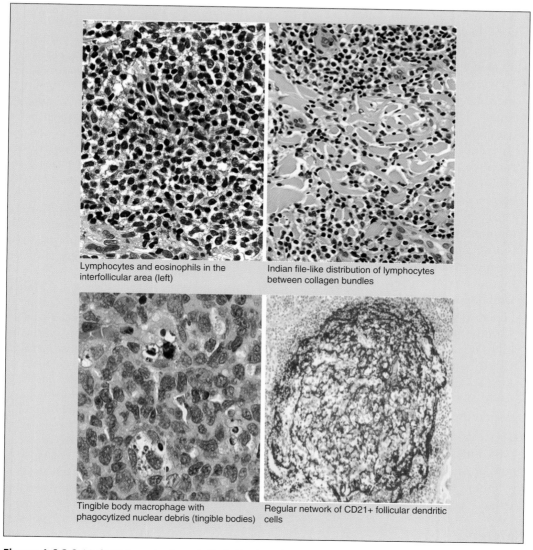

Lymphocytes and eosinophils in the interfollicular area (left)

Indian file-like distribution of lymphocytes between collagen bundles

Tingible body macrophage with phagocytized nuclear debris (tingible bodies)

Regular network of CD21+ follicular dendritic cells

Figure 1.6.2.2 Variant: Lymphadenosis Cutis Benigna (Pseudolymphoma; Lymphocytoma Cutis) (Stage I).
Source: Burg et al. (2019). *Atlas of Dermatopathology: Tumors, Nevi, and Cysts* (p. 394). Oxford: Wiley.

In Europe, in a minority of cases pseudolymphomatous infiltrates most commonly occur some weeks after infection with *Borrelia burgdorferi* at the site of a previous tick bite (*Ixodes ricinus*).

CF: Mostly solitary, rarely multiple or disseminated soft red, sharply bordered nodules on the head, preferentially on the ear lobes. Other predilection sites are the nose, nipples, inguinal area, and the scrotum.

HF: Nodular dermal infiltrates, mainly located in the upper and mid-dermis, occasionally extending into the deep dermis.

- Preserved subepidermal grenz zone
- Dense and diffuse lymphoid infiltrates
- Reactive lymph follicles

- Follicle centers with "starry sky"-pattern: macrophages containing phagocytosed nuclear material (Fleming's tingible body macrophages)
- Follicle centers with large (centroblasts) and small (centrocytes) follicle center cells
- Small lymphocytes around reactive lymph follicles
- Interfollicular area composed of small B-cells, diffusely splayed small T-cells, histiocytes, and a few eosinophils and plasma cells
- Characteristically, there is diffuse splaying of round cells between collagen or smooth muscle bundles (e.g. at the nipple), subsequently creating the impression of smudging borders – whereas cutaneous B-cell lymphoma typically presents with sharply demarcated borderlines
- Immunophenotype: Polyclonal B-cell infiltrate; monotypic expression of kappa or lambda chains is exceptional. Regular and sharply demarcated network of CD21+ follicular dendritic cells within the reactive lymph follicles

DD: Cutaneous B-cell lymphomas (marginal zone lymphoma; follicle center lymphoma); other pseudolymphomas caused by other microbiological, physical, or chemical agents.

Reference

Braun-Falco, O. B., & Burg, G. (1975). [Lymphoreticular proliferations in the skin. Cytochemical and immunocytological studies in lymphadenosis benigna cutis]. *Hautarzt*, **26**(3), 124–132.

Baefverstedt, B. (1944). Ueber lymphadenosis benigna cutis. Eine klinische pathologisch-anatomische Studie. *Acta Derm Venereol (Suppl XI) (Stockh)*, **24**, 1–102.

Buechner, S. A., Lautenschlager, S., Itin, P., Bircher, A., & Erb, P. (1995). Lymphoproliferative responses to Borrelia burgdorferi in patients with erythema migrans, acrodermatitis chronica atrophicans, lymphadenosis benigna cutis, and morphea. *Arch Dermatol*, **131**(6), 673–677.

Colli, C., Leinweber, B., Mullegger, R., Chott, A., Kerl, H., & Cerroni, L. (2004). Borrelia burgdorferi-associated lymphocytoma cutis: Clinicopathologic, immunophenotypic, and molecular study of 106 cases. *J Cutan Pathol*, **31**(3), 232–240.

Grange, F., Wechsler, J., Guillaume, J. C., Tortel, J., Tortel, M. C., Audhuy, B., . . . Cerroni, L. (2002). Borrelia burgdorferi-associated lymphocytoma cutis simulating a primary cutaneous large B-cell lymphoma. *J Am Acad Dermatol*, **47**(4), 530–534.

Moulonguet, I., Ghnassia, M., Molina, T., & Fraitag, S. (2012). Miliarial-type perifollicular B-cell pseudolymphoma (lymphocytoma cutis): A misleading eruption in two women. *J Cutan Pathol*, **39**(11), 1016–1021.

Rijlaarsdam, J. U., Meijer, C. J., & Willemze, R. (1990). Differentiation between lymphadenosis benigna cutis and primary cutaneous follicular center cell lymphomas. A comparative clinicopathologic study of 57 patients. *Cancer*, **65**(10), 2301–2306.

Watanabe, R., Nanko, H., & Fukuda, S. (2006). Lymphocytoma cutis due to pierced earrings. *J Cutan Pathol*, **33**(Suppl 2), 16–19.

1.6.3 Variant: Morphea/Scleroderma-Like Lesions (Stage II)

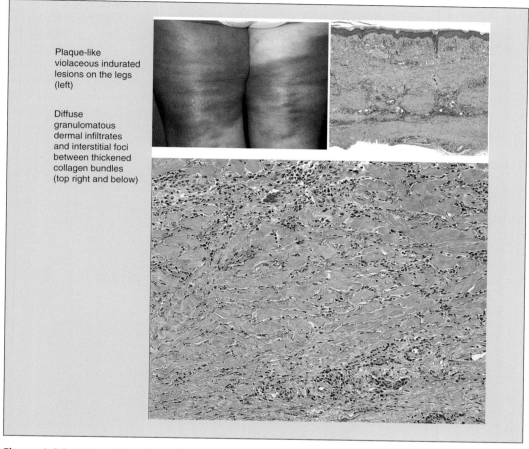

Plaque-like violaceous indurated lesions on the legs (left)

Diffuse granulomatous dermal infiltrates and interstitial foci between thickened collagen bundles (top right and below)

Figure 1.6.3 Variant: Morphea/Scleroderma-Like Lesions (Stage II).

Plaque-like erythematous indurations which closely resemble early morphea/scleroderma – occasionally presenting with edematous and granulomatous infiltrates (early stages).

CF: A few weeks following prior ECM manifestation, plaque-like indurated lesions develop at the site of the resolving ECM. Clinical and histopathological differential diagnoses of early stages (lilac ring) comprise interstitial granulomatous dermatitis, interstitial granulomatous drug reaction, morphea/scleroderma (lilac ring), and granuloma annulare (diffuse type).

HF:
- Diffuse granulomatous dermal infiltrates, with characteristic splaying of tiny granulomatous interstitial foci, often spilling over into the upper subcutis
- Multiple tiny wreath-like granulomas ("micro-rosettes") with telltale free-floating thickened collagen bundles at the center and pale histiocytes at the periphery
- Additionally, throughout the entire dermis sparse diffuse mixed infiltrate, often containing histiocytes, eosinophils, and plasma cells

- Preserved elastic fiber network; no scarring

DD: Remarkably, a similar – if not identical – histopathological pattern (biopsy taken from inflamed periphery/lilac ring) may be encountered in morphea/scleroderma, interstitial granulomatous dermatitis (in conjunction with rheumatoid arthritis or with other autoimmune disorders), and interstitial granulomatous drug reactions.

Reference

Aberer, E., Klade, H., Stanek, G., & Gebhart, W. (1991). Borrelia burgdorferi and different types of morphea. *Dermatologica*, **182**(3), 145–154.

Breier, F., Khanakah, G., Stanek, G., Kunz, G., Aberer, E., Schmidt, B., & Tappeiner, G. (2001). Isolation and polymerase chain reaction typing of Borrelia afzelii from a skin lesion in a seronegative patient with generalized ulcerating bullous lichen sclerosus et atrophicus. *Br J Dermatol*, **144**(2), 387–392.

Breier, F. H., Aberer, E., Stanek, G., Khanakaha, G., Schlick, A., & Tappeiner, G. (1999). Isolation of Borrelia afzelii from circumscribed scleroderma. *Br J Dermatol*, **140**(5), 925–930.

Wackernagel, A., Bergmann, A. R., & Aberer, E. (2005). Acute exacerbation of systemic scleroderma in Borrelia burgdorferi infection. *J Eur Acad Dermatol Venereol*, **19**(1), 93–96.

1.6.4 Variant: Acrodermatitis Chronica Atrophicans (Stage III)

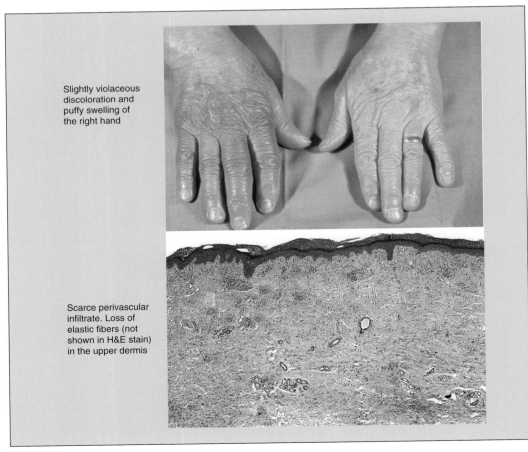

Slightly violaceous discoloration and puffy swelling of the right hand

Scarce perivascular infiltrate. Loss of elastic fibers (not shown in H&E stain) in the upper dermis

Figure 1.6.4.1 Variant: Acrodermatitis Chronica Atrophicans (Stage III).

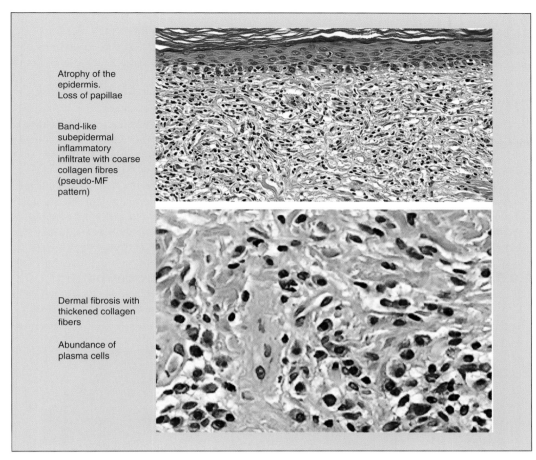

Figure 1.6.4.2 Variant: Acrodermatitis Chronica Atrophicans (Stage III).

CF: In stage II of borreliosis (usually months or years after infection) – preferentially on the limbs, mostly unilaterally, rarely bilaterally – a violaceous puffy edema appears that gradually evolves into cutaneous atrophy ("cigarette paper-type" skin, telangiectasias, red-brownish color) with characteristically translucent superficial blood vessels. Fibrosis and sclerosis with scleroderma-like collagen changes, ulnar and tibial fibro-sclerotic bands, and juxta-articular fibrous (fibroid) nodules are accompanying features of advanced acrodermatitis chronica atrophicans.

HF:

- Dermal edema and mucin deposits (early)
- Markedly thinned, atrophied epidermis (late)
- Loss of rete ridges and cutaneous adnexa (late)
- Dilated superficial blood vessels (early and late)
- Diffuse superficial round cell infiltrate, hugging the epidermis ("pseudo-MF")
- Additional perivascular infiltrates, superficial and deep, with conspicuous plasma cells
- Dense, diffuse interstitial round cell infiltrate with abundant plasma cells (late)
- Rarely, adjacent paucicellular fibroid nodules surrounded by abundant plasma cells at periphery (late)

Remarkably, in some cases of advanced Borrelia infection, T-cell rich infiltrates composed of small T-cells with or without plasma cells develop that may mimic mycosis fungoides ("Pseudo-MF" pattern of borreliosis) both clinically and histologically.

DD: Anetoderma; atrophoderma of Pasini and Pierini; varicose veins; actinic reticuloid – with histopathological morphological overlap, albeit clinically completely different.

Reference

Gulseren, D., Cerroni, L., Hofmann-Wellenhof, R., & Arzberger, E. (2018). Correlation of reflectance confocal microscopy and dermatopathology findings in a case of Acrodermatitis chronica atrophicans. *Am J Dermatopathol*, **40**(5), 367–370.

Kempf, W., Kazakov, D. V., Hubscher, E., Gugerli, O., Gerbig, A. W., Schmid, R., . . . Kutzner, H. (2015). Cutaneous borreliosis associated with T cell-predominant infiltrates: A diagnostic challenge. *J Am Acad Dermatol*, **72**(4), 683–689.

Tee, S. I., Martinez-Escaname, M., Zuriel, D., Fried, I., Wolf, I., Massone, C., & Cerroni, L. (2013). Acrodermatitis chronica atrophicans with pseudolymphomatous infiltrates. *Am J Dermatopathol*, **35**(3), 338–342.

Zalaudek, I., Leinweber, B., Kerl, H., & Mullegger, R. R. (2005). Acrodermatitis chronica atrophicans in a 15-year-old girl misdiagnosed as venous insufficiency for 6 years. *J Am Acad Dermatol*, **52**(6), 1091–1094.

1.6.5 Variant: Juxta-Articular Fibrous Nodules in Acrodermatitis Chronica Atrophicans (Stage III)

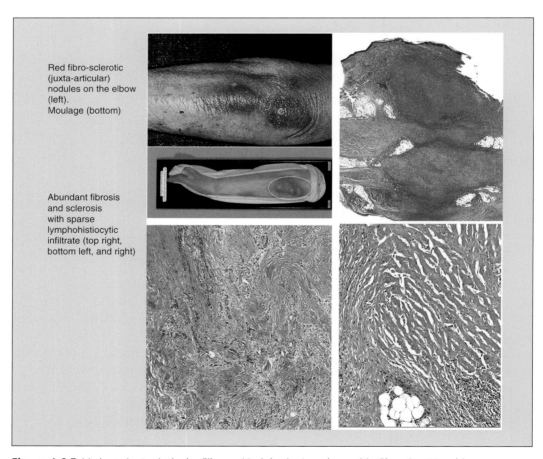

Red fibro-sclerotic (juxta-articular) nodules on the elbow (left). Moulage (bottom)

Abundant fibrosis and sclerosis with sparse lymphohistiocytic infiltrate (top right, bottom left, and right)

Figure 1.6.5 Variant: Juxta-Articular Fibrous Nodules in Acrodermatitis Chronica Atrophicans (Stage III).

CF: Reddish to violaceous juxta-articular subcutaneous nodules, preferentially close to the elbows, often with concomitant translucent atrophic skin. Remarkably hard consistency ("wood-hard" nodules).
HF: Lamellated compact paucicellular fibrosis and sclerosis, with abundant polyclonal plasma cells at its outer fringes.
DD: Rheumatoid nodule; dermatofibroma; keloid and hypertrophic scar; erythema elevatum diutinum (advanced stage).

Reference

Espana, A., Torrelo, A., Guerrero, A., Suarez, J., Rocamora, A., & Ledo, A. (1991). Periarticular fibrous nodules in Lyme borreliosis. *Br J Dermatol*, **125**(1), 68–70.

Messer, L., Felten, R., Moreau, P., Freisz, M. C., & Mahe, A. (2015). Fibrous nodules over the patella revealing acrodermatitis chronica atrophicans. *Joint Bone Spine*, **82**(3), 208.

Netherton, E. W., & Hubler, W. R. (1945). Acrodermatitis atrophicans chronica with fibrous cutaneous nodules. *Arch Derm Syphilol*, **52**, 416.

1.6.6 Differential Diagnosis: Actinic Reticuloid°

UV-light induced disorder; often idiopathic or associated with sensitizing chemical agents.

CF: Clinically, there is remarkable thickening and coarse wrinkling of the skin, almost exclusively at sun-exposed sites (face).
HF: There may be slight morphological overlap with the incipient stage of borreliosis.

- Parakeratosis, acanthosis, spongiosis
- Dermal dendrocytes and multinucleated giant cells
- Lichenoid lymphocytic infiltrate, containing many plasma cells and eosinophils
- Fibrosis

DD: Borreliosis; cutaneous T-cell lymphoma; eczema, persistent light reaction; phototoxic and photoallergic dermatitis.

Reference

Sidiropoulos, M., Deonizio, J., Martinez-Escala, M. E., Gerami, P., & Guitart, J. (2014). Chronic actinic dermatitis/actinic reticuloid: A clinicopathologic and immunohistochemical analysis of 37 cases. *Am J Dermatopathol*, **36**(11), 875–881.

Toonstra, J., Henquet, C. J., van Weelden, H., van der Putte, S. C., & van Vloten, W. A. (1989). Actinic reticuloid. A clinical photobiologic, histopathologic, and follow-u study of 16 patients. *J Am Acad Dermatol*, **21**(2 Pt 1), 205–214.

1.7 Venereal Diseases

1.7.1 Gonorrhea

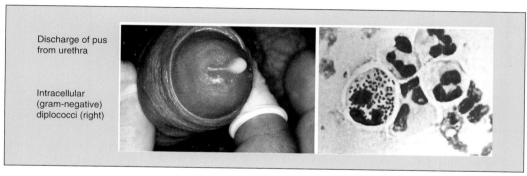

Discharge of pus from urethra

Intracellular (gram-negative) diplococci (right)

Figure 1.7.1 Gonorrhea.

CF: Burning sensation of urethra in conjunction with pus-laden discharge. Associated systemic ("benign") gonococcal sepsis may occur in rare cases (see chapter on sepsis).

HF: Direct identification of bacteria in smears, showing intracellular gram-negative diplococci. Supportive diagnostic methods: Immunofluorescence, culture, PCR (urine, smear, biopsy).

DD: Non-gonococcal urethritis.

1.7.2 Syphilis, Chancre

Treponema pallidum infection is acquired mostly via direct sexual contact. Classically, untreated syphilis evolves through three well-defined clinicopathological stages. Remarkably, at each stage syphilis may mimic various non-venereal diseases. Conversely, inflammatory dermatoses of various origin may show morphological overlap with *Treponema pallidum* infection, for example, pustular psoriasis and pustular stage II of syphilis.

Reference

Borroni, G. (1988). A case of late congenital syphilis at the Metropolitan Museum of Art, New York. *Am J Dermatopathol*, **10**(5), 448–450.

Ober, W. B. (1989). To cast a pox. The iconography of syphilis. *Am J Dermatopathol*, **11**(1), 74–86.

1.7.2.1 Stage I

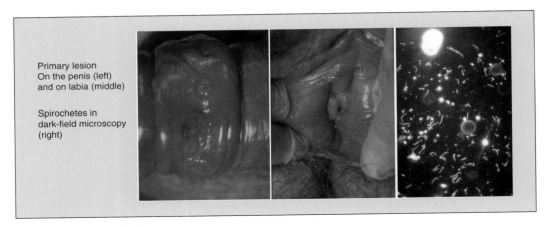

Primary lesion
On the penis (left)
and on labia (middle)

Spirochetes in
dark-field microscopy
(right)

Figure 1.7.2.1 Syphilis (Stage I).

CF: After an incubation period of about 2–3 weeks, ulcus durum (chancre) – the first visible manifestation of *T. pallidum* infection – develops at the primary site of infectious entry, typically at the penis (sulcus coronarius), vulva, cervix uteri, perianal skin, lips, or oral cavity. The ulcer is painless; there is always associated regional lymphadenitis.

At this early stage of disease, diagnosis can be established by the direct demonstration of spirochetes (smears; dark field microscopy) and by serological tests, which become reactive/positive 2–3 weeks after primary infection (specific IgM antibodies).

HF:

- Shallow ulceration, often with serum and debris
- Accompanying edema
- Dense mixed inflammatory infiltrate
- Abundant plasma cells
- Dilated postcapillary venules with swelling of endothelial cells

- Histopathological demonstration of *Treponema pallidum* by Warthin–Starry silver stain and/or immunohistochemically

DD: Non-infectious balanitis plasmacellularis Zoon; chancroid of *Haemophilus ducreyi* infection.

Reference

Carlson, J. A., Dabiri, G., Cribier, B., & Sell, S. (2011). The immunopathobiology of syphilis: The manifestations and course of syphilis are determined by the level of delayed-type hypersensitivity. *Am J Dermatopathol*, **33**(5), 433–460.

1.7.2.2 Stage II

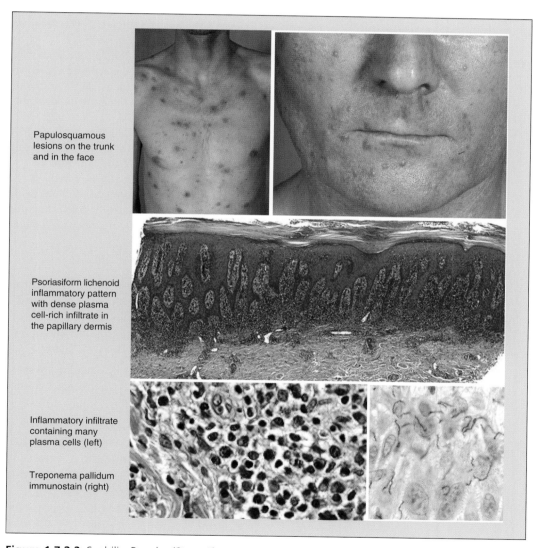

Papulosquamous lesions on the trunk and in the face

Psoriasiform lichenoid inflammatory pattern with dense plasma cell-rich infiltrate in the papillary dermis

Inflammatory infiltrate containing many plasma cells (left)

Treponema pallidum immunostain (right)

Figure 1.7.2.2 Syphilis, Papular (Stage II).
Source: Burg et al. (2019). *Atlas of Dermatopathology: Tumors, Nevi, and Cysts* (p. 398). Oxford: Wiley.

CF: In the early secondary stage of syphilis (8–12 weeks after infection), distinct tiny macules (roseola) may appear on trunk and extremities, that are easily overlooked and regress spontaneously. In the late stage of secondary syphilis (>2 years after untreated infection), disseminated small papules and papulosquamous lesions may appear on head, trunk, extremities, and on mucous membranes, presenting as plaques and patches on the palms and soles ("pustular psoriasis") or as condyloma-like lesions in the anogenital region.

HF:

- Macular lesions: Nonspecific sparse interstitial infiltrate; few plasma cells as a telltale sign of infectious origin
- Maculopapular lesions in late secondary syphilis
  - Interface dermatitis; often associated with spongiosis with subcorneal spongiform pustulation
  - Dermal edema
  - Superficial and deep perivascular and interstitial infiltrate
  - Mixed infiltrate: lymphocytes, histiocytes, mostly scattered – occasionally numerous – eosinophils
  - Sheets or small focal clusters of plasma cells – as a clue to the diagnosis
  - Histiocyte-predominant granulomatous features at advanced stages
  - Spirochetes may be detected either by Warthin–Starry silver stain or immunohistochemically, preferentially in the upper dermis and epidermis
- Verruciform condylomata lata – with markedly spongiform pustulation – and ulcerating lues maligna – with broad shallow ulcers and massive debris – are variants of secondary syphilis at special sites, preferentially in immunocompromised patients. Spirochetes may be abundant in these conditions

DD: Pityriasis lichenoides et varioliformis acuta (PLEVA); pustular psoriasis; lymphomatoid papulosis; cutaneous lymphoma (mycosis fungoides); drug reaction; tick bites; leprosy.

Reference

Alessi, E., Innocenti, M., & Ragusa, G. (1983). Secondary syphilis. Clinical morphology and histopathology. *Am J Dermatopathol*, **5**(1), 11–17.

Jordaan, H. F. (1988). Secondary syphilis. A clinicopathological study. *Am J Dermatopathol*, **10**(5), 399–409.

Pettit, C., McMurray, S., Randall, M. B., Jones, A., & Fisher, K. (2019). Highlighting a potential pitfall: Positive Treponema pallidum immunohistochemical stain in a patient without syphilis. *Am J Dermatopathol*, **41**(12), 924–926.

Rosa, G., Bennett, D., & Piliang, M. P. (2015). Eosinophil-rich syphilis: A report of four cases. *J Cutan Pathol*, **42**(8), 554–558.

Rysgaard, C., Alexander, E., & Swick, B. L. (2014). Nodular secondary syphilis with associated granulomatous inflammation: Case report and literature review. *J Cutan Pathol*, **41**(4), 370–379.

1.7.2.3 Stage III°

CF: Two years after primary infection, the course of disease – provided there was no appropriate treatment – reaches its third, latent stage. Clinical symptoms are manifold: gummatous superficial or deep ulcerating skin lesions, cardiovascular (aorta), peripheral and central neurologic symptoms (progressive paralysis, tabes dorsalis).

HF:

- Small granulomas composed of epithelioid cells and multinucleated giant cells
- Lymphohistiocytic infiltrates with plasma cells
- Dilated vessels with swollen endothelia
- Central caseating necrosis

DD: Sarcoidosis; tuberculosis; leprosy; leishmaniasis (advanced).

1.7.3 Ulcus Molle (Chancroid)

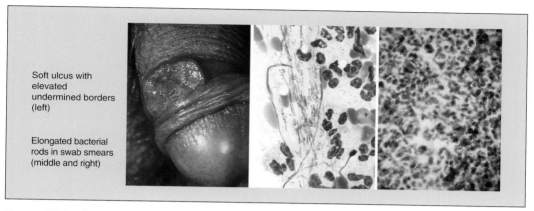

Soft ulcus with elevated undermined borders (left)

Elongated bacterial rods in swab smears (middle and right)

Figure 1.7.3 Ulcus Molle (Chancroid).

Haemophilus ducreyi is a gram-negative rod-like bacterium that infects the skin or mucous membranes via small superficial injuries.

CF: The most frequent sites of primary infection are the female labia majora and minora and the inner fold of the foreskin in men. The initial papule evolves into a painful ulcer with elevated undermined borders, from which a diagnostic smear may be taken for microscopic investigation.

HF: Smears taken from the base of the ulcus or its borders reveal large numbers of *Haemophilus ducreyi,* arranged in long chains.

DD: Other ulcerating venereal disease; herpes genitalis.

Reference

Freinkel, A. L. (1987). Histological aspects of sexually transmitted genital lesions. *Histopathology*, **11**(8), 819–831.

King, R., Gough, J., Ronald, A., Nasio, J., Ndinya-Achola, J. O., Plummer, F., & Wilkins, J. A. (1996). An immunohistochemical analysis of naturally occurring chancroid. *J Infect Dis*, **174**(2), 427–430.

1.7.4 Granuloma Inguinale (Donovanosis; Granuloma Venereum)

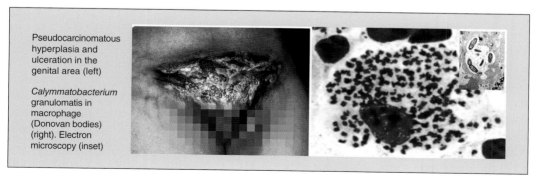

Pseudocarcinomatous hyperplasia and ulceration in the genital area (left)

Calymmatobacterium granulomatis in macrophage (Donovan bodies) (right). Electron microscopy (inset)

Figure 1.7.4 Granuloma Inguinale (Donovanosis; Granuloma Venereum).

Granuloma inguinale is caused by the gram-negative bacterium *Klebsiella granulomatis (Calymmatobacterium granulomatis)*. Granuloma inguinale (syn: granuloma venereum) is not to be confused with **lympho**granuloma inguinale (syn: **lympho**granuloma venereum), which is a venereal infection caused by *Chlamydia trachomatis*.

CF: Small papules evolving into chronically progressive painless ulcers, preferentially at the male genitalia; mostly in tropical and subtropical regions. Ulcers with characteristically hypertrophic lateral borders. Concomitant lymphadenopathy is usually absent.

HF:

- Pseudocarcinomatous epithelial hyperplasia at the outer border of the ulcer
- Central ulceration with prominent necrosis
- Diffuse inflammatory infiltrate, containing macrophages, plasma cells, and neutrophils
- Macrophages with intracytoplasmic inclusion (Donovan bodies)
- Demonstration of bacterial rods in semithin sections (toluidine blue or Giemsa stain)

DD: Ulcus mole (chancroid); ulcus durum (syphilis); herpes simplex/genitalis.

1.7.5 Lymphogranuloma Inguinale (Lymphogranuloma Venereum; Duran-Nicolas–Favre Disease)

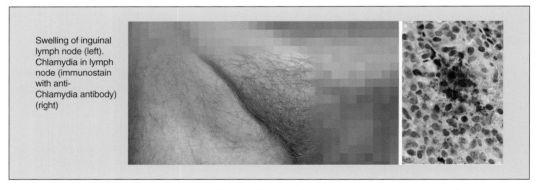

Swelling of inguinal lymph node (left). Chlamydia in lymph node (immunostain with anti-Chlamydia antibody) (right)

Figure 1.7.5 Lymphogranuloma Inguinale (Lymphogranuloma Venereum; Durand–Nicolas–Favre Disease).

This sexually transmitted infection caused by *Chlamydia trachomatis* should not be confused with another, sound-alike venereal infection – granuloma inguinale (syn: granuloma venereum) – which is caused by the gram-negative bacterium *Calymmatobacterium granulomatis*.

CF: Primary lesion (stage I) is an ulcerating papulopustule, usually in the genital region or in the rectum. In stage II, the regional lymph node is involved (bubo), which shows abscess formation with ulceration and draining to the surface. Stricture and fibrosis in stage III (elephantiasis) eventually evolve into massive lymphatic edema and urethral-vaginal fistulas.

HF: Unspecific findings with ulceration and granulomatous abscess formation.

Fibrosis and scarring at later stages. The lymph nodes show granulomatous inflammation with many plasma cells and abscess formation. Chlamydia organisms preferentially are demonstrated by immunohistochemical methods (specific monoclonal antibodies).

DD: Syphilis; granuloma inguinale; herpes simplex/genitalis; other genital ulcers.

1.8 Rickettsial Infections

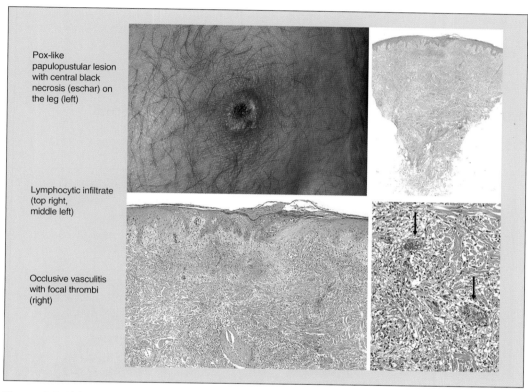

Pox-like papulopustular lesion with central black necrosis (eschar) on the leg (left)

Lymphocytic infiltrate (top right, middle left)

Occlusive vasculitis with focal thrombi (right)

Figure 1.8 Rickettsial Infections.

Rickettsiae comprise a family of gram-negative intracellular parasites (Rickett-siaceae family), which are transmitted by various vectors (ticks, mites, flees, lice) and cause spotted fever, endemic typhus, Rocky Mountain spotted fever, Mediterranean tick fever, African tick bite fever, Rickettsial pox, and others. The different rickettsial diseases are subsumed under various groups: spotted fevers-group, typhus group, and others – in particular, Q-fever, where the vector is not an arthropod; infectious organisms are inhaled.

CF: Diffuse exanthema – often associated with fever and chills – or solitary papulo-pustular lesion with marked central necrosis and hemorrhagic crust; the central eschar is highly characteristic. Occasional swelling of the draining lymph node. Milder forms may be associated with itching sensation.

HF: Histologic changes of solitary lesion, for example, in Mediterranean tick fever:

• Flat ulcer with superficial necrosis and crust formation (eschar)
• Superficial and deep perivascular infiltrate
• Focal leukocytoclastic vasculitis with small thrombi (telltale sign)
• Organisms may be demonstrated immunohistochemically or by immunofluorescence. Rickettsiae often thrive within the walls of small inflamed vessels

DD: Mosquito bite; furuncle; leishmaniasis; ecthyma; orf; anthrax (solitary lesion with eschar).

Reference

Montenegro, M. R., Mansueto, S., Hegarty, B. C., & Walker, D. H. (1983). The histology of "taches noires" of boutonneuse fever and demonstration of Rickettsia conorii in them by immunofluorescence. *Virchows Arch A Pathol Anat Histopathol*, **400**(3), 309–317.

1.9 Dermatoses Associated with Bacterial Infections

1.9.1 Staphylococcal Scalded Skin Syndrome (SSSS)

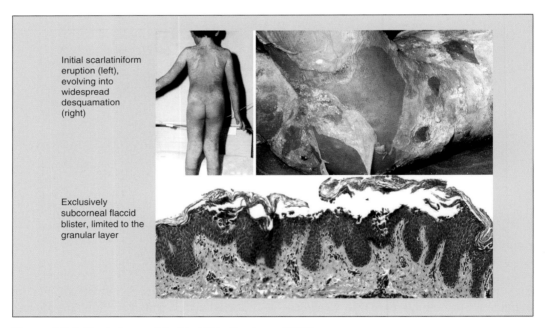

Initial scarlatiniform eruption (left), evolving into widespread desquamation (right)

Exclusively subcorneal flaccid blister, limited to the granular layer

Figure 1.9.1 Staphylococcal Scalded Skin Syndrome (SSSS).

Also known as dermatitis exfoliativa neonatorum, Ritter [von Rittershain] disease, staphylococcal Lyell syndrome, Pemphigus neonatorum.

Toxin-mediated epidermolytic dermatosis, primarily in small children, characterized by erythema and widespread loss of the superficial epidermal layers, resembling acute burn. Causative agent is the toxin-producing (exfoliative toxins A and B) *Staphylococcus aureus*, often of phage group II.

CF: Initially, there is a mild scarlatiniform rash with associated fever. Widespread erythema evolves into marked tenderness with small unstable flaccid bullae that quickly erode and lead to burn-like loss of superficial epithelial layers. The clinical course often is acute with systemically ill patients.

HF:

• Subcorneal acantholysis and blister formation with a marked split high in the epidermis
• Blister roof composed exclusively of stratum corneum (versus blister formation in TEN, where full-thickness epidermal blister roof occurs)
• Little or no inflammatory infiltrate

• Frozen sections preferred for rapid diagnosis

DD: Toxic epidermal necrolysis (TEN) showing full-thickness epidermal detachment.

Reference

Cribier, B., Piemont, Y., & Grosshans, E. (1994). Staphylococcal scalded skin syndrome in adults. A clinical review illustrated with a new case. *J Am Acad Dermatol*, **30**(2 Pt 2), 319–324.

de Dobbeleer, G., & Achten, G. (1975). Staphylococcal scalded skin syndrome. *An ultrastructural study. J Cutan Pathol*, **2**(2), 91–98.

Elston, D. M., Stratman, E. J., & Miller, S. J. (2016). Skin biopsy: Biopsy issues in specific diseases. *J Am Acad Dermatol*, **74**(1), 1–16.

1.9.2 Differential Diagnosis: Toxic Epidermal Necrolysis (TEN)

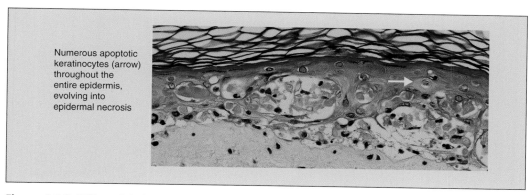

Numerous apoptotic keratinocytes (arrow) throughout the entire epidermis, evolving into epidermal necrosis

Figure 1.9.2 Differential Diagnosis: Toxic Epidermal Necrolysis (TEN).

Severe immunological drug-induced (in particular, antibiotic and antiepileptic drugs) skin reaction, characterized by complete epidermal necrosis (keratinocyte necrosis) and associated mucosal involvement.

CF: Incipient confluent maculopapular exanthem, followed by hemorrhagic blisters and widespread epidermal necrosis resulting in wide denuded areas of skin. Positive Nikolski's sign. Massive periorificial mucosal erosions are common.

HF: At early stages, scatter of necrotic keratinocytes throughout the epidermis.

Advanced lesions with full-thickness epidermal necrosis. Necrotic epidermis often completely detached from underlying cutis. The inflammatory infiltrate may be very sparse (versus erythema multiforme and fixed drug eruption with marked interface dermatitis). Frozen sections should be preferred for rapid histopathological diagnosis.

DD: Staphylococcal scaled skin syndrome (with flaccid subcorneal bullae); acute burns; erythema multiforme; fixed drug eruption; pemphigus and pemphigoid variants; linear IgA disease.

Reference

Naik, H., Lockwood, S., & Saavedra, A. (2017). A pilot study comparing histological and immunophenotypic patterns in stage 4 skin graft vs host disease from toxic epidermal necrolysis. *J Cutan Pathol*, **44**(10), 857–860.

Ondhia, C., Kaur, C., Mee, J., Natkunarajah, J., & Singh, M. (2019). Lichen planus pemphigoides mimicking toxic epidermal necrolysis. *Am J Dermatopathol*, **41**(11), e144–147.

Paquet, P., & Pierard, G. E. (1997). Erythema multiforme and toxic epidermal necrolysis: A comparative study. *Am J Dermatopathol*, **19**(2), 127–132.

Schwartz, R. A., McDonough, P. H., & Lee, B. W. (2013). Toxic epidermal necrolysis: Part I. Introduction, history, classification, clinical features, systemic manifestations, etiology, and immunopathogenesis. *J Am Acad Dermatol*, **69**(2): 173.e1–13; quiz 185–6.

1.10 Dermatoses Mimicking Bacterial Infections

1.10.1 Pyoderma Gangrenosum

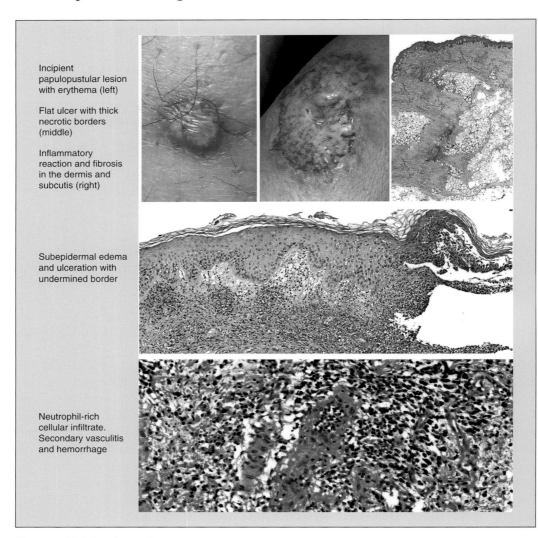

Figure 1.10.1 Pyoderma Gangrenosum.

The key pathogenetic process in the uncommon disorder bearing the misnomer "pyoderma gangrenosum" is a massive suppurative infiltration with neutrophils and associated vessel damage. PG and Sweet syndrome are paradigmatic autoinflammatory disorders and should be evaluated and treated under this particular etiopathogenetic concept. PG frequently is associated with inflammatory bowel disease (colitis ulcerosa), rheumatoid arthritis, autoinflammatory disorders, hepatitis or occurs as a sequela to traumatic or surgical wounds in patients with a distinctive predisposition to PG.

CF: Typically, banal postoperative or traumatic wounds rapidly enlarge, and evolve with centrifugally expanding erythema into a central pustular or bullous eruption with subsequent fulminant ulceration. Ulcers show pathognomonically undermined borders with necrosis and hemorrhage. The lower leg is the preferential site. Multiple lesions may coalesce. Lesions resolve from the center, leaving typical cribriform scars.

Variants of PG include bullous, superficial granulomatous, pustular vegetative, peristomal, genital, and postoperative types. Remarkably, PG may show a plethora of different histopathological patterns. Diagnosis therefore should always be based on strict clinic-pathological correlation!

HF:

- Incipient (unspecific) suppurative "folliculitis," followed by shallow ulcer formation
- Shallow ulcer with undermined borders
- Subepidermal edema evolving into diffuse neutrophil-rich infiltrate
- Predominantly neutrophilic infiltrate, accompanied by few lymphocytes, plasma cells, and histiocytes. Morphological overlap with Sweet syndrome-like pattern
- Secondary vasculitis with intraluminal fibrin deposits and neutrophils
- End stage of PG with deep-reaching (unspecific) ulceration involving the subcutaneous fat

DD: Ecthyma; artifact; deep fungal or bacterial infection.

Reference

Azar, M. M., Relich, R. F., Schmitt, B. H., Spech, R. W., & Hage, C. A. (2014). Cutaneous blastomycosis masquerading as pyoderma gangrenosum. *J Clin Microbiol*, **52**(4), 1298–1300.

Saunderson, R. B., Tng, V., Watson, A., & Scurry, J. (2016). Perianal herpes simplex virus infection misdiagnosed with Pyoderma gangrenosum: Case of the month from the Case Consultation Committee of the International Society for the Study of Vulvovaginal Disease. *J Low Genit Tract Dis*, **20**(2), e14–15.

1.10.2 Infantile Acropustulosis

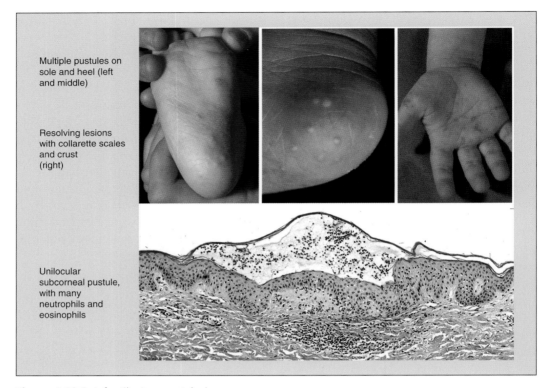

Multiple pustules on sole and heel (left and middle)

Resolving lesions with collarette scales and crust (right)

Unilocular subcorneal pustule, with many neutrophils and eosinophils

Figure 1.10.2 Infantile Acropustulosis.

CF: At birth or during the first year of life, pruritic pustules with an erythematous base occur on hands and feet, resolving with collarette-type scale-crusts, in most cases within two years. Unknown etiology.

HF:

• Unilocular, subcorneal or intraepidermal vesicle or pustule
• Sparse spongiosis at the periphery of the lesion
• Pustules contain a mixed round cell infiltrate, with predominant neutrophils and eosinophils

• Bacteria or fungi are not demonstrable with special stains

DD: Scabies; impetigo; pustular psoriasis; acrodermatitis continua suppurativa Hallopeau; IgA bullous dermatosis; IgA pemphigus.

Reference

Hürlimann, A., Wüthrich, B., & Burg, G. (1992). Infantile Akropustulose. *Z Hautkr*, **67**(12), 1073–1079.
Paloni, G., Berti, I., & Cutrone, M. (2013). Acropustulosis of infancy. *Arch Dis Child Fetal Neonatal Ed*, **98**(4), F340.

1.10.3 Acute Generalized Exanthematous Pustulosis (AGEP)

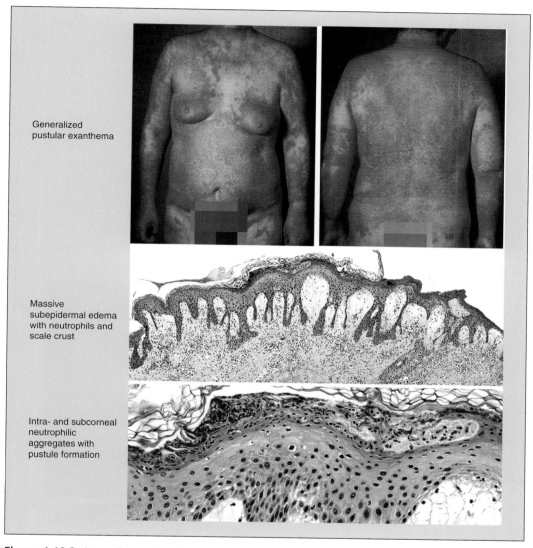

Generalized pustular exanthema

Massive subepidermal edema with neutrophils and scale crust

Intra- and subcorneal neutrophilic aggregates with pustule formation

Figure 1.10.3 Acute Generalized Exanthematous Pustulosis (AGEP).

Most eruptions of AGEP are caused by antibiotic drugs. Historically, mercury has played a significant role in some cases.

CF: Sudden eruption of myriads of small pustules on erythematous ground, combined with fever and leukocytosis.

HF:

- Superficial intra- or subcorneal pustule, filled with neutrophils
- Spongiosis at the margin of the lesion
- Edema of the papillary dermis
- Sparse mixed cellular inflammatory infiltrate in the upper and deep dermis

- Almost always erythrocyte extravasation
- Leukocytoclastic vasculitis may be present (facultative)

DD: Pustular psoriasis; Sweet syndrome; Sneddon–Wilkinson syndrome; impetigo; **D**rug **R**ash with **E**osinophilia and **S**ystemic **S**ymptoms (DRESS); leukocytoclastic vasculitis; incipient stage of erysipelas.

Reference

Ballmer, B. K., Widmer, M., & Burg, G. (1993). Acetylsalicylsäure-induzierte generalisierte Pustulose. *Schweiz med Wschr*, **123**, 542–546.

Poeschl, M. D., Hurley, M. Y., Goyal, S. D., & Vidal, C. I. (2014). Targetoid eruptions: Acute generalized exanthematous pustulosis. *Am J Dermatopathol*, **36**(10), 827–828, 838.

Sidoroff, A., Halevy, S., Bavinck, J. N., Vaillant, L., & Roujeau, J. C. (2001). Acute generalized exanthematous pustulosis (AGEP) – a clinical reaction pattern. *J Cutan Pathol*, **28**(3), 113–119.

Vyas, N. S., Charifa, A., Desman, G. T., & McNiff, J. M. (2019). Distinguishing pustular psoriasis and acute generalized exanthematous pustulosis on the basis of plasmacytoid dendritic cells and MxA protein. *J Cutan Pathol*, **46**(5), 317–326.

1.10.4 Psoriasis Pustulosa

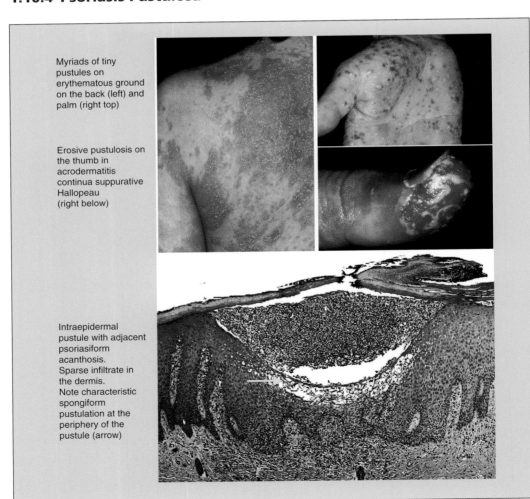

Myriads of tiny pustules on erythematous ground on the back (left) and palm (right top)

Erosive pustulosis on the thumb in acrodermatitis continua suppurative Hallopeau (right below)

Intraepidermal pustule with adjacent psoriasiform acanthosis. Sparse infiltrate in the dermis. Note characteristic spongiform pustulation at the periphery of the pustule (arrow)

Figure 1.10.4 Psoriasis Pustulosa.

CF: Generalized pustular psoriasis (von Zumbusch type) is characterized by generalized eruption of aggregated tiny pustules, densely grouped pustular lesions on a macular erythema, and associated fever and malaise.

Acrodermatitis continua suppurativa (Hallopeau) is a localized clinical variant of psoriasis pustulosa at acral sites, mostly on the fingers and toes.

HF:

- Acanthosis and papillomatosis, slightly psoriasiform, often with accompanying scale crust
- Pathognomonic "spongiform pustulation": Subcorneal pustules, filled with neutrophils, and neutrophil-rich spongiosis at the edges of the lesion – corresponding to Kogoj's "unicellular pustule"
- Spongiform changes at the bottom and at the outer edges may predominate in early lesions

- Sparse to moderate predominantly neutrophilic infiltrate in the dermis
- No infectious organisms

DD: Pustular drug reaction; impetigo contagiosa.

Reference

Kardaun, S. H., Kuiper, H., Fidler, V., & Jonkman, M. F. (2010). The histopathological spectrum of acute generalized exanthematous pustulosis (AGEP) and its differentiation from generalized pustular psoriasis. *J Cutan Pathol*, **37**(12), 1220–1229.

Sanchez, N. P., Perry, H. O., & Muller, S. A. (1981). On the relationship between subcorneal pustular dermatosis and pustular psoriasis. *Am J Dermatopathol*, **3**(4), 385–386.

Vyas, N. S., Charifa, A., Desman, G. T., & McNiff, J. M. (2019). Distinguishing pustular psoriasis and acute generalized exanthematous pustulosis on the basis of plasmacytoid dendritic cells and MxA protein. *J Cutan Pathol*, **46**(5), 317–326.

1.10.5 Localized Neutrophilic Eccrine Hidradenitis Associated with Mitoxantrone Treatment

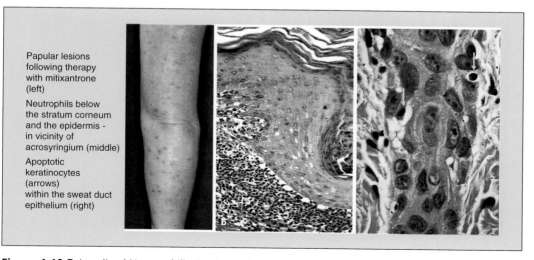

Papular lesions following therapy with mitixantrone (left)

Neutrophils below the stratum corneum and the epidermis - in vicinity of acrosyringium (middle)

Apoptotic keratinocytes (arrows) within the sweat duct epithelium (right)

Figure 1.10.5 Localized Neutrophilic Eccrine Hidradenitis.

CF: In this self-limited disorder, which frequently is a sequela to treatment with anthracyclines, multiple small firm reddish sweat-gland-bound papules or pustules appear on the limbs or on the trunk. Underlying hematologic or other malignancies (treatment) are almost always present.

HF:

- Predominantly neutrophilic round cell infiltrate next to or within the subepidermal acrosyringeal portion of the eccrine (and apocrine) sweat ducts
- Sweat glands and duct epithelium may show only minor vacuolization and

occasional apoptosis; complete necrosis does not occur

DD: Other chemotherapy-induced drug eruptions

Reference

Brehler, R., Reimann, S., Bonsmann, G., & Metze, D. (1997). Neutrophilic hidradenitis induced by chemotherapy involves eccrine and apocrine glands. *Am J Dermatopathol*, **19**(1), 73–78.

Burg, G., Bieber, T., & Lanecker, P. (1988). Lokalisierte neutrophile ekkrine Hidradenitis unter Mitoxantron: Eine typische Zytostatikanebenwirkung. *Hautarzt*, **39**, 233–236.

1.10.6 Erosive Pustular Dermatitis (Pustular Ulcerative Dermatosis) of the Scalp

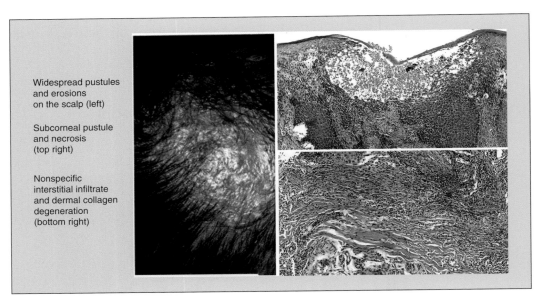

Widespread pustules and erosions on the scalp (left)

Subcorneal pustule and necrosis (top right)

Nonspecific interstitial infiltrate and dermal collagen degeneration (bottom right)

Figure 1.10.6 Erosive Pustular Dermatitis of the Scalp.

Rare disease of unknown etiology, primarily seen in elderly patients. A nosologic relationship with pyoderma gangrenosum has been suggested.

CF: Crusty erosions and pustules on the scalp.

HF: Erosive pustular dermatitis of the scalp may mimic a plethora of superficial erosive dermatoses in sun-damaged skin. Histopathological changes are often misleading:

- Subcorneal pustules (early) – often in association with actinic keratosis
- Flat erosion evolving into shallow ulcer with slightly hyperplastic borders (late)
- Accompanying massive actinic elastosis and solar keratosis (telltale signs)
- Neutrophil-rich diffuse infiltrate without vasculitis and without demonstrable infectious organisms

DD: Subcorneal pustular dermatosis (Sneddon–Wilkinson); pyoderma gangrenosum; primary or secondary bacterial or fungal infection of the scalp; IgA pemphigus (advanced).

Reference

Bieber, T., Ruzicka, T., & Burg, G. (1987). Erosive pustulöde Dermatitis des Kapillitiums. *Hautarzt*, **38**, 687–689.

Starace, M., Loi, C., Bruni, F., Alessandrini, A., Misciali, C., Patrizi, A., & Piraccini, B. M. (2017). Erosive pustular dermatosis of the scalp: Clinical, trichoscopic, and histopathologic features of 20 cases. *J Am Acad Dermatol.* 2017 Jun;76(6):1109–1114.e2.

Tomasini, C., & Michelerio, A. (2019). Erosive pustular dermatosis of the scalp: A neutrophilic folliculitis within the spectrum of neutrophilic dermatoses: A clinicopathologic study of 30 cases. *J Am Acad Dermatol*, **81**(2), 527–533.

CHAPTER 2

Fungal Infections

CHAPTER MENU

2.1 Superficial Cutaneous Fungal Infections
   2.1.1 Variants: Tinea Corporis; Tinea Faciei
   2.1.2 Variants: Tinea Barbae; Tinea Capitis (Trichophytia)
   2.1.3 Granuloma Trichophyticum (Majocchi's Granuloma)
   2.1.4 Candidiasis (Moniliasis)
   2.1.5 Candida Tropicalis and Candida Lipolytica
   2.1.6 Pityriasis (Tinea) Versicolor
   2.1.7 Variant: Malassezia (Pityrosporum) Folliculitis
   2.1.8 Differential Diagnosis: Seborrheic Dermatitis
   2.1.9 Tinea Nigra
   2.1.10 Piedra (Trichomycosis Nodosa Alba and Nigra)°
2.2 Subcutaneous Mycoses
   2.2.1 Sporotrichosis
   2.2.2 Mycetoma (Madura Foot)
   2.2.3 Chromo(blasto)mycosis (Dermatitis Verrucosa)

2.3 Systemic Mycoses (Deep Fungal Infections)
   2.3.1 Cryptococcosis (Torulosis, European Blastomycosis)
   2.3.2 North American Blastomycosis (Blastomycosis, Chicago Disease)
   2.3.3 Lobomycosis (Lobo Disease, Keloidal Blastomycosis, Blastomycoid Granuloma)
   2.3.4 Histoplasmosis
   2.3.5 Coccidioidomycosis (Desert or Valley Fever, San Joaquin Fever)
   2.3.6 Paracoccidioidomycosis (South American Blastomycosis)
   2.3.7 Emmonsiosis
2.4 Opportunistic Fungal Infections
   2.4.1 Aspergillosis (Alternaria)
   2.4.2 Zygomycosis (Mucormycosis; Phycomycosis)
   2.4.3 Hyalohyphomycosis
   2.4.4 Phaeohyphomycosis
   2.4.5 Prototothecosis, Cutaneous

°no pictures

Atlas of Clinical Dermatopathology: Infectious and Parasitic Dermatoses, First Edition. Günter Burg, Heinz Kutzner, Werner Kempf, Josef Feit, and Omar Sangueza.
© 2021 John Wiley & Sons Ltd. Published 2021 by John Wiley & Sons Ltd.

Reference

Hibbett, D. S., Binder, M., Bischoff, J. F., Blackwell, M., Cannon, P. F., Eriksson, O. E., . . . Zhang, N. (2007). A higher-level phylogenetic classification of the Fungi. *Mycol Res*, **111**(Pt 5), 509–547.

2.1 Superficial Cutaneous Fungal Infections

Fungi comprise a very large number of species ("the kingdom of fungi"). The taxonomy of fungi differentiates divisions, subdivisions, classes, and subclasses. Only a minority of these fungal species is clinically relevant in humans. Fungi with pathogenic potential for the skin are classified into three categories:

1. Dermatophytes, including *Microsporum, Epidermophyton*, and *Trichophyton* (growing with hyphae, which are multicellular filaments)
2. Yeasts (eukaryotic single-celled microorganisms)
3. Molds (growing with hyphae, which are multicellular filaments)

Identification and classification of fungi traditionally is done with the help of special culture media, or by PCR (ITS1 and ITS2), with the latter method being faster and much more precise.

From a dermatological and practical point of view, fungal infections are best classified into superficial and deep types. Established clinical nomenclature prefers the prefix "tinea" with the appropriate suffix, naming the infected anatomic structure or site, for example, tinea corporis, tinea barbae, tinea manuum, tinea pedum. Deviant terminology referring to the pathogenic species or to the distinct anatomic structures is also used in exceptional cases.

As this is not a review of mycology, in the following the clinical and histopathologic features of the most common cutaneous fungal infections are displayed irrespective of their taxonomic orders.

Reference

Gupta, A. K., Chaudhry, M., & Elewski, B. (2003). Tinea corporis, tinea cruris, tinea nigra, and piedra. *Dermatol Clin*, **21**(3), 395–400.

Gupta, A. K., Ryder, J. E., Nicol, K., & Cooper, E. A. (2003). Superficial fungal infections: An update on pityriasis versicolor, seborrheic dermatitis, tinea capitis, and onychomycosis. *Clin Dermatol*, **21**(5), 417–425.

Schwartz, R. A. (2004). Superficial fungal infections. *Lancet*, **364**(9440), 1173–1182.

2.1.1 Variants: Tinea Corporis; Tinea Faciei

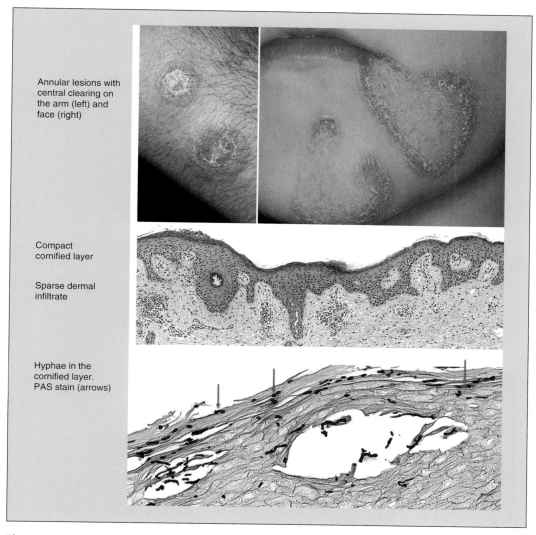

Annular lesions with central clearing on the arm (left) and face (right)

Compact cornified layer

Sparse dermal infiltrate

Hyphae in the cornified layer. PAS stain (arrows)

Figure 2.1.1 Variants: Tinea Corporis; Tinea Faciei.
Source: Burg et al. (2015). *Atlas of Dermatopathology: Practical Differential Diagnosis by Clinicopathologic Pattern* (p. 75). Oxford: Wiley.

The term "tinea" in conjunction with the site of infection (tinea corporis, capitis, barbae, manus, pedis, inguinalis) commonly characterizes a cutaneous infection with dermatophytes. As always in dermatology, there are confusing "sound-alike" exceptions of nomenclature with no nosological relationship to classic fungal infection at all, for example, tinea (taenia) amiantacea, which is a bacterial infection. Clinical features largely depend on the anatomic site (glabrous or non-glabrous skin, intertriginous sites, mucous membranes). Tinea corporis is the prototypical infection with dermatophytes.

CF: Small pustules, crusts and scaling with centrifugal growth, and tendency to regression in the center of the circumscribed lesions ("tinea" = ringworm).

HF:

- Compact orthokeratosis with prominent scales, albeit very little serum exudate ("hyphae do not swim")
- Neutrophilic granulocytes within corneal layer as a pathognomonic sign ("neuts in the horn")
- Neutrophil-predominant dermal infiltrate
- Hyphae and spores often in or around hair shaft within hair follicle (tinea profunda)
- PAS stain demonstrates hyphae and spores, and therefore is mandatory for all neutrophilic dermatoses

DD: Eczema; lichen planus.

Reference

Kash, N., Ginter-Hanselmayer, G., & Cerroni, L. (2010). Cutaneous mycotic infections with pseudolymphomatous infiltrates. *Am J Dermatopathol*, **32**(5), 514–517.

Miedema, J. R., Merritt, B., & Zedek, D. (2012). Dermatophyte infection resembling a lichen planus-like keratosis. *J Cutan Pathol*, **39**(9), 889–890.

Meymandi, S., Silver, S. G., & Crawford, R. I. (2003). Intraepidermal neutrophils – a clue to dermatophytosis? *J Cutan Pathol*, **30**(4), 253–255.

2.1.2 Variants: Tinea Barbae; Tinea Capitis (Trichophytia)

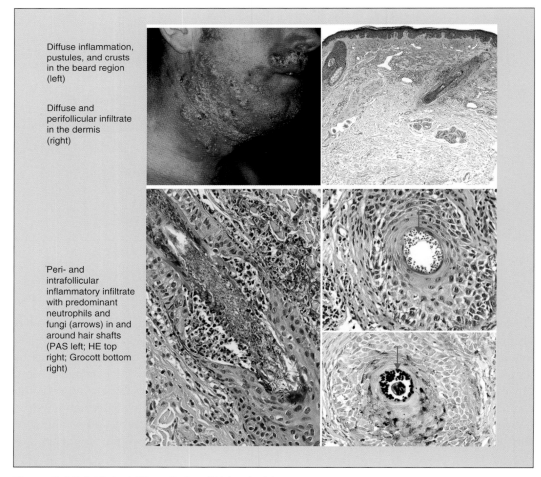

Diffuse inflammation, pustules, and crusts in the beard region (left)

Diffuse and perifollicular infiltrate in the dermis (right)

Peri- and intrafollicular inflammatory infiltrate with predominant neutrophils and fungi (arrows) in and around hair shafts (PAS left; HE top right; Grocott bottom right)

Figure 2.1.2.1 Variant: Tinea Barbae (Trichophytia).

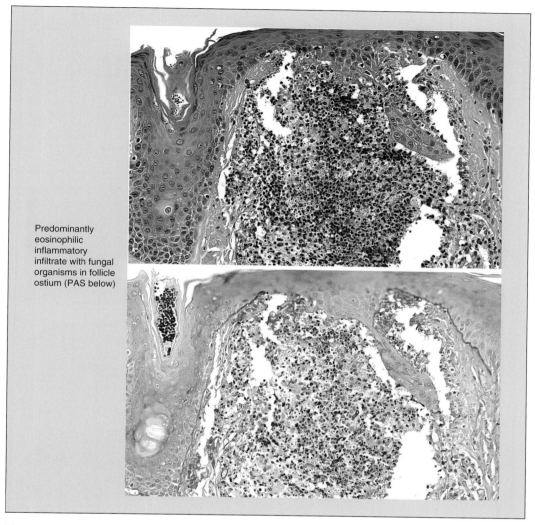

Predominantly eosinophilic inflammatory infiltrate with fungal organisms in follicle ostium (PAS below)

Figure 2.1.2.2 Variant: Tinea Barbae (Trichophytia).

Fungal infection of the hair. Tinea favosa (favus) is an endemic variant due to infection by *Trichophyton schoenleinii*, mostly on the head of children.

CF: Inflammatory plaques and infiltration of the skin with pustules, crusts, and (temporary) hair loss.

HF:

- Neutrophil-predominant mixed inflammatory infiltrate throughout the dermis
- Hair follicle with neutrophils and incipient abscess formation
- Follicular and perifollicular debris and granulomatous infiltrate (late)

- Hyphae and spores within (endotrich) and around (exotrich) the hair shaft

DD: Eczema; bacterial folliculitis; alopecia areata; lichen planopilaris; mucinosis follicularis.

Reference

Amer, M., Helmy, A., & Amer, A. (2017). Trichoscopy as a useful method to differentiate tinea capitis from alopecia areata in children at Zagazig University Hospitals. *Int J Dermatol*, **56**(1), 116–120.

El-Taweel, A. E., El-Esawy, F., & Abdel-Salam, O. (2014). Different trichoscopic features of tinea capitis and alopecia areata in pediatric patients. *Dermatol Res Pract*, **2014**, 848763.

Kirsten, H., Haiduk, J., Nenoff, P., Uhrlass, S., Ziemer, M., & Simon, J. C. (2019). [Tinea barbae profunda due to Trichophyton mentagrophytes:

Case report and review]. *Hautarzt*, **70**(8), 601–611.

Singh, S., Sondhi, P., Yadav, S., & Ali, F. (2017). Tinea barbae presenting as kerion. *Indian J Dermatol Venereol Leprol*, **83**(6), 741.

2.1.3 Granuloma Trichophyticum (Majocchi's Granuloma)

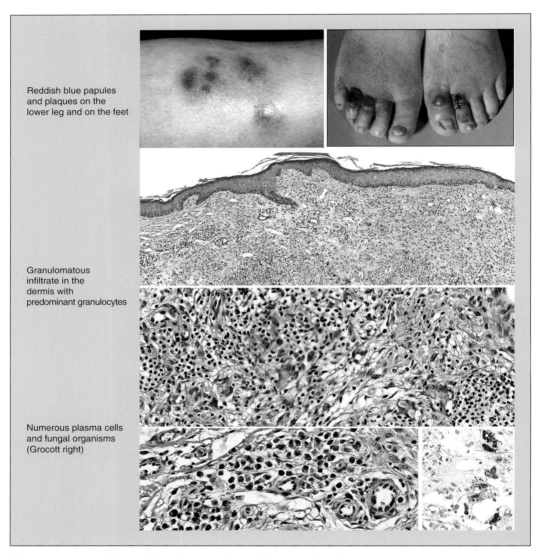

Reddish blue papules and plaques on the lower leg and on the feet

Granulomatous infiltrate in the dermis with predominant granulocytes

Numerous plasma cells and fungal organisms (Grocott right)

Figure 2.1.3 Granuloma Trichophyticum (Majocchi's Granuloma).

Granulomatous reaction following follicular infection with dermatophytes, often combined with granulomatous perifollicular foreign body reaction; preferentially on lower legs of women (secondary to hair shaving of the legs).

DD: Other granulomatous infections, for example, granulomatous folliculitis and granulomatous rosacea.

Reference

Kaneko, T., & Kaneko, M. (2017). A patient with cystic granuloma trichophyticum who required surgical resection. *Med Mycol J*, **58**(1), E29–E32.

Nishiyama, C., Miyaji, M., & Morioka, S. (1983). A case of generalized granuloma trichophyticum. *Mycopathologia*, **82**(2), 77–82.

2.1.4 Candidiasis (Moniliasis)

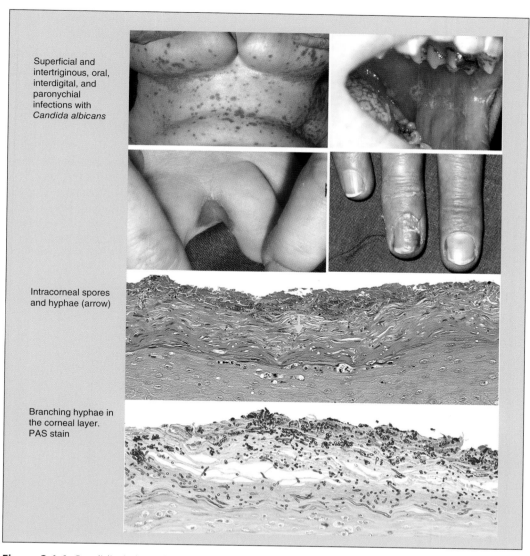

Superficial and intertriginous, oral, interdigital, and paronychial infections with *Candida albicans*

Intracorneal spores and hyphae (arrow)

Branching hyphae in the corneal layer. PAS stain

Figure 2.1.4 Candidiasis (Moniliasis).

Candidiasis is an originally harmless commensal colonization with opportunistic yeasts of the genus *Candida* which in the presence of predisposing factors (diabetes, obesity, corticosteroids, antibiotic therapy, immunosuppression, malnutrition, severe illness) has evolved into a long-lasting cutaneous infection of mucous membranes or skin. Most candida infections are caused by *Candida albicans*, which is a common organism in the autochthonous microbiome of the oral cavity, gastrointestinal tract, and external genitalia. Apart from *C. albicans*, there are several other candida species which – less frequently – may be pathogenetic.

CF: Pruritic erythema, erosions, rhagades, maceration and easily removable whitish plaques of the mucous membranes. Underlying granulomas or pustules and folliculitis may present various clinical pictures, depending on the site of infection. Sites of predilection are the oral and genital mucosa, the large skin folds, the interdigital and intertriginous areas, and nails with their paronychia.

HF:

- Thick hyphae and pseudo-hyphae (induced by repeated budding) and spores in the upper corneal layer (PAS)
- Hyperkeratosis, focal parakeratosis, and papillomatosis (late)
- Mixed inflammatory infiltrate in the upper dermis
- Granulomatous changes with multinucleated giant cells may be present in chronic variants
- Mucous membranes of the oral cavity often show secondary candidiasis overlying leukoplakia and squamous cell carcinoma

DD: Eczema; psoriasis; lichen planus on the mucosa; stomatitis and glossitis geographica; bacterial infections; pityriasis versicolor

Reference

Hauser, F. V., & Rothman, S. (1950). Monilial granuloma; report of a case and review of the literature. *Arch Derm Syphilol*, **61**(2), 297–310.

Kugelman, T. P., Cripps, D. J., & Harrell, E. R., Jr. (1963). Candida granuloma with epidermophytosis. Report of a case and review of the literature. *Arch Dermatol*, **88**, 150–157.

2.1.5 Candida Tropicalis and Candida Lipolytica

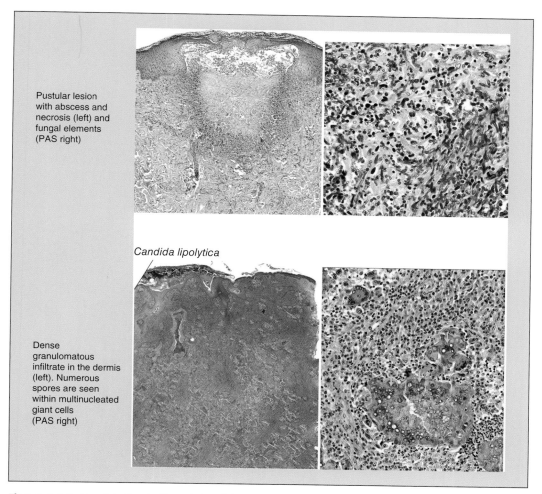

Pustular lesion with abscess and necrosis (left) and fungal elements (PAS right)

Candida lipolytica

Dense granulomatous infiltrate in the dermis (left). Numerous spores are seen within multinucleated giant cells (PAS right)

Figure 2.1.5 Candida Tropicalis and Candida Lipolytica.

These are rare mostly systemic infections, seen preferentially in neutropenic or immunocompromised patients.

Reference

Benson, P. M., Roth, R. R., & Hicks, C. B. (1987). Nodular subcutaneous abscesses caused by Candida tropicalis. *J Am Acad Dermatol*, **16**(3 Pt 1), 623–624.

Walsh, T. J., Salkin, I. F., Dixon, D. M., & Hurd, N. J. (1989). Clinical, microbiological, and experimental animal studies of Candida lipolytica. *J Clin Microbiol*, **27**(5), 927–931.

2.1.6 Pityriasis (Tinea) Versicolor

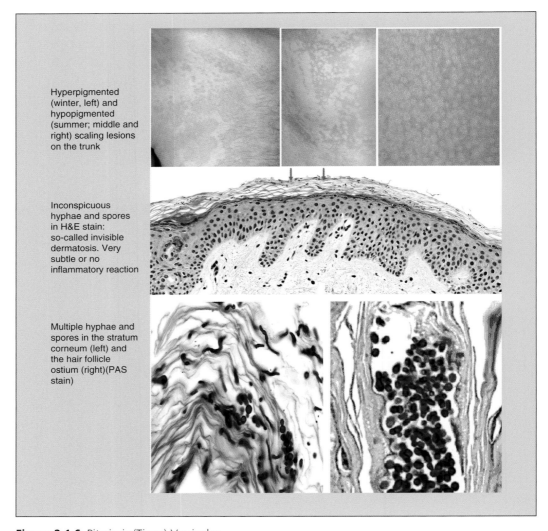

Hyperpigmented (winter, left) and hypopigmented (summer; middle and right) scaling lesions on the trunk

Inconspicuous hyphae and spores in H&E stain: so-called invisible dermatosis. Very subtle or no inflammatory reaction

Multiple hyphae and spores in the stratum corneum (left) and the hair follicle ostium (right)(PAS stain)

Figure 2.1.6 Pityriasis (Tinea) Versicolor.

The dimorphic lipophilic yeast *Malassezia furfur* (*Pityrosporum ovale* or *orbiculare*) is part of the normal skin flora and presents with varying phenotypes. Hyphae and spores may regularly be found in the follicle ostia. Massive expansion of *Malassezia* colonies preferentially affects young adults during summer months, mostly in humid climates, with hyperhidrosis and occlusive dressing, but also immunocompromised patients with subfebrile body temperature (telltale sign). Pityriasis versicolor is a result of the yeast's transformation from a saprophytic form in healthy skin to a pathogenic mycelial form in diseased skin. Azelaic acid, which is produced by the yeasts, blocks melanin synthesis and serves as a blanching agent, which in conjunction with the UV-shielding effect of the overlying scales at affected sites accounts for the changes in skin color: whitish in the summer and brownish in the winter.

CF: Small, sharply demarcated hypo- or hyperpigmented leaf-like or geographical patches with discrete pityriasiform scaling, preferentially on the trunk.

HF:

- Inconspicuous, regular skin at scanning magnification ("invisible dermatosis")
- Compact orthokeratosis
- Numerous PAS-positive hyphae and spores ("spaghetti and meatballs")
- Very scant inflammatory infiltrate in the upper dermis, suggesting diagnosis of vitiligo
- The marked discrepancy between the large number of fungal elements and the scant accompanying inflammatory infiltrate is characteristic for pityriasis versicolor

DD: Seborrheic dermatitis; pityriasis rosea; postinflammatory hyper- or hypo-pigmentation; pityriasis alba in young patients with atopy; vitiligo (no scaling).

Reference

Gupta, A. K., Batra, R., Bluhm, R., Boekhout, T., & Dawson, T. L., Jr. (2004). Skin diseases associated with Malassezia species. *J Am Acad Dermatol*, **51**(5), 785–798.

Veerappan, R., Miller, L. E., Sosinski, C., & Youngberg, G. A. (2006). Narrow-spectrum staining pattern of Pityrosporum. *J Cutan Pathol*, **33**(11), 731–734.

2.1.7 Variant: Malassezia (Pityrosporum) Folliculitis

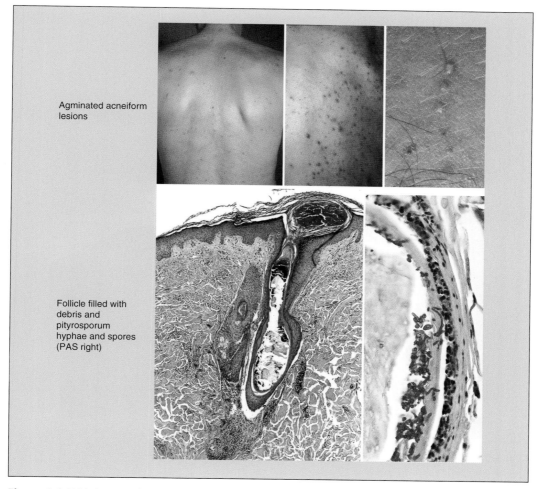

Agminated acneiform lesions

Follicle filled with debris and pityrosporum hyphae and spores (PAS right)

Figure 2.1.7 Variant: Malassezia (Pityrosporum) Folliculitis.

Infection of hair follicles, preferentially in immunocompromised patients.

CF: Monomorphic eruption of small acneiform lesions, mostly on the trunk.

HF:

- *Malassezia furfur*, hyphae and spores, within follicle and follicle ostium
- Dense perifollicular infiltrate with predominant neutrophils
- Neutrophils in follicular wall
- Perifollicular debris and granulomatous infiltration (late)

DD: Acne; "Mallorca acne"; other forms of infectious and non-infectious folliculitis; neonatal cephalic pustulosis.

Reference

Clemmensen, O. J., & Hagdrup, H. (1991). Splendore-Hoeppli phenomenon in Pityrosporum folliculitis (pseudoactinomycosis of the skin). *J Cutan Pathol*, **18**(4), 293–297.

Sina, B., Kauffman, C. L., & Samorodin, C. S. (1995). Intrafollicular mucin deposits in Pityrosporum folliculitis. *J Am Acad Dermatol*, **32**(5 Pt 1), 807–809.

2.1.8 Differential Diagnosis: Seborrheic Dermatitis

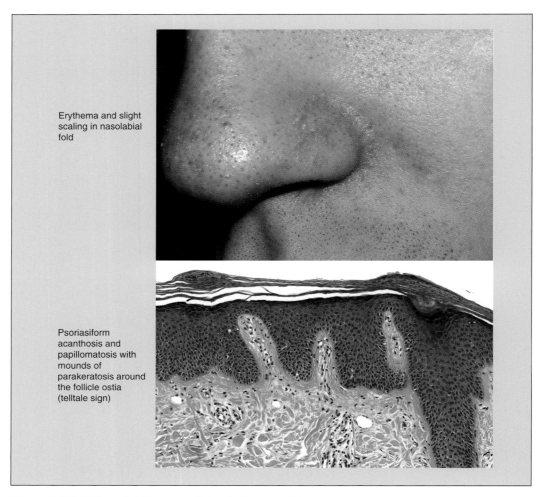

Erythema and slight scaling in nasolabial fold

Psoriasiform acanthosis and papillomatosis with mounds of parakeratosis around the follicle ostia (telltale sign)

Figure 2.1.8 Differential Diagnosis: Seborrheic dermatitis.
Source: Burg et al. (2015). *Atlas of Dermatopathology: Practical Differential Diagnosis by Clinicopathologic Pattern* (p. 55). Wiley.

CF: Erythema and scaling, preferentially in the centrofacial area, breast, scalp.

HF: Psoriasiform acanthosis and hyperparakeratosis overlying hair follicle ostia, exocytosis of neutrophils.

2.1.9 Tinea Nigra

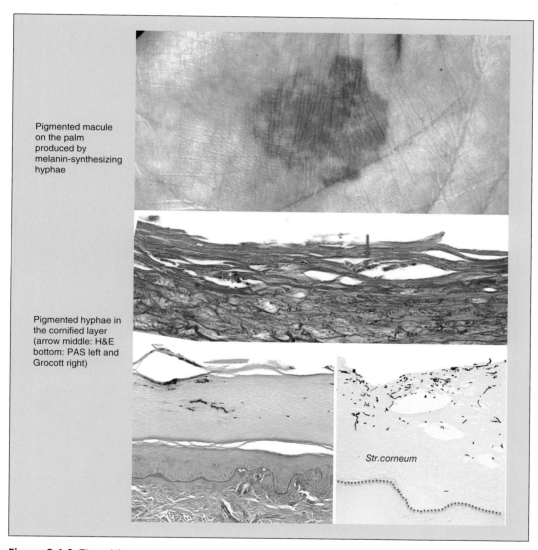

Pigmented macule on the palm produced by melanin-synthesizing hyphae

Pigmented hyphae in the cornified layer (arrow middle: H&E bottom: PAS left and Grocott right)

Str.corneum

Figure 2.1.9 Tinea Nigra.

Superficial mycotic infection by the geophilic and dematiaceous mold *Hortaea werneckii* (formerly *Exophiala werneckii*).

CF: Preferentially in tropical climates, a circumscribed asymptomatic lentiginous hyperpigmentation occurs on the soles, rarely on the palms. Clinically diagnosis is usually missed as the lesions appear to be of melanocytic origin.

HF: Elongated empty spaces and gaps within the thickened cornified layer, often associated with cloudy whitish foci where PAS stain may show pigmented hyphae and spores. Although *Hortaea werneckii* is a melanin-producing fungus, immunohistochemical stains with antimelanocytic antibodies (HMB45) are usually negative.

2.1.10 Piedra (Trichomycosis Nodosa Alba and Nigra)°

Piedra (Spanish "stone") is an asymptomatic superficial fungal infection of the hair shaft. The black variant of piedra is caused by *Piedraia hortae* (a mold) in tropical areas; the white variant usually is caused by *Trichosporon asahii*.

_____
°no pictures

CF: Tiny firm nodules, attached to the hairs of the scalp (black piedra) or the axillae, the pubes, beard, and eyebrows (white piedra).

HF: Diagnosis is made clinically.

DD: Trichobacteriosis (trichomycosis) palmellina; nits; hair casts; hair shaft anomalies like trichorrhexis nodosa.

2.2 Subcutaneous Mycoses

2.2.1 Sporotrichosis

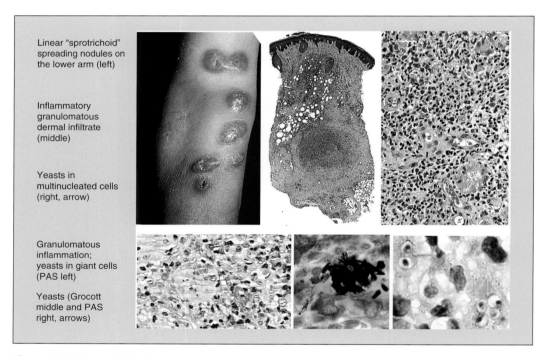

Linear "sprotrichoid" spreading nodules on the lower arm (left)

Inflammatory granulomatous dermal infiltrate (middle)

Yeasts in multinucleated cells (right, arrow)

Granulomatous inflammation; yeasts in giant cells (PAS left)

Yeasts (Grocott middle and PAS right, arrows)

Figure 2.2.1 Sporotrichosis.

Sporothrix schenckii is a saprophytic dimorphic fungus. Percutaneous inoculation from soil or wood occurs mostly by trauma.

CF: Cutaneous and subcutaneous firm nodules, spreading from the inoculation site in a moniliform pattern ("sporotrichoid spreading") along lymphatics, from where the infectious process can disseminate into adjacent soft tissue. Nodules often ulcerate.

HF:
- Inflammatory dermal granulomatous infiltrate
- *Sporotrichon* within the cytoplasm of large, multinucleated histiocytes (PAS)
- Many plasma cells and neutrophils
- Asteroid bodies in 40% of specimens
- In cases with ulceration, pseudocarcinomatous epithelial hyperplasia at the outer fringes of the lesion

DD: Other deep fungal and mycobacterial infections, leprosy, syphilis, leishmaniasis.

Reference

Quintella, L. P., Passos, S. R., do Vale, A. C., Galhardo, M. C., Barros, M. B., Cuzzi, T., . . . Schubach Ade, O. (2011). Histopathology of cutaneous sporotrichosis in Rio de Janeiro: A series of 119 consecutive cases. *J Cutan Pathol*, **38**(1), 25–32.

Rodriguez, G., & Sarmiento, L. (1998). The asteroid bodies of sporotrichosis. *Am J Dermatopathol*, **20**(3), 246–249.

Zhang, Y. Q., Xu, X. G., Zhang, M., Jiang, P., Zhou, X. Y., Li, Z. Z., & Zhang, M. F. (2011). Sporotrichosis: Clinical and histopathological manifestations. *Am J Dermatopathol*, **33**(3), 296–302.

2.2.2 Mycetoma (Madura Foot)

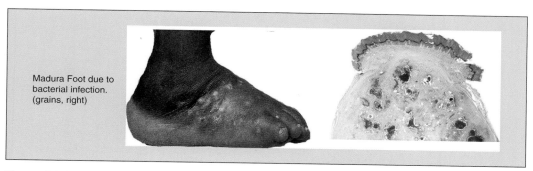

Madura Foot due to bacterial infection. (grains, right)

Figure 2.2.2 Mycetoma (Madura Foot).

Mycetoma is an uncommon chronic infection of skin and subcutaneous tissues in tropical countries. Percutaneous inoculation by various eumycotic fungi, which thrive mostly in soil, or by *Actinomyces* (bacteria), produces chronic, localized infection of the skin and the subcutaneous tissue, often involving adjacent muscle and bone. A definite histopathological and microbiological examination is mandatory because the treatment may be entirely different.

CF: Massive erythematous disfiguring edema and swelling, preferentially on the foot, with discharge of white or yellow grains via broad sinuses.

HF:

- Chronic fibrosing inflammation
- Grains of the causative fungi or bacteria (PAS, Gram, or silver stain)

DD: Chronic fibrosing swelling and inflammation due to various causes; actinomycosis.

Reference

Alam, K., Maheshwari, V., Bhargava, S., Jain, A., Fatima, U., & Haq, E. U. (2009). Histological diagnosis of madura foot (mycetoma): A must for definitive treatment. *J Glob Infect Dis*, **1**(1), 64–67.

2.2.3 Chromo(blasto)mycosis (Dermatitis Verrucosa)

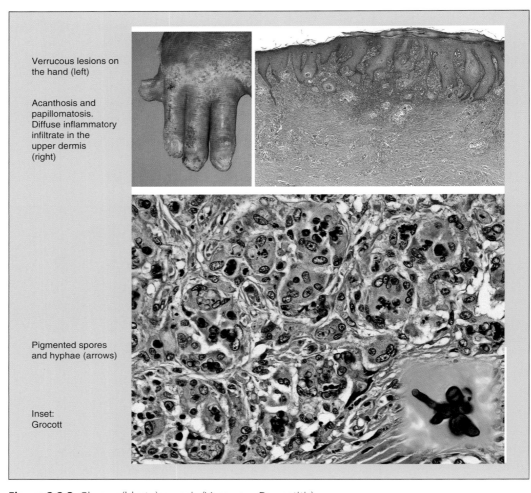

Verrucous lesions on the hand (left)

Acanthosis and papillomatosis. Diffuse inflammatory infiltrate in the upper dermis (right)

Pigmented spores and hyphae (arrows)

Inset: Grocott

Figure 2.2.3 Chromo(blasto)mycosis (Verrucous Dermatitis).

Several darkly pigmented fungi that thrive in soil and in decaying wood, mostly in tropical and subtropical areas, cause chromoblastosis. Sites of predilection are the feet where infection occurs mostly via banal superficial wounds. Five organisms are responsible for most cases: *Fonsecaea pedrosoi, Phialophora verrucosa, Fonsecaea compacta, Cladosporium carrionii*, and *Rhinocladiella aquaspersa*.

CF: At the site of inoculation – mostly the feet – a slowly growing papule occurs,

evolving into a papillomatous plaque with verrucous hyperkeratosis. These lesions may enlarge to wide verrucous plaques, covering most of the foot.

HF:

- Acanthosis and papillomatosis
- Variable hyperkeratosis, often associated with marked pseudocarcinomatous hyperplasia
- Granulomatous infiltrate in the dermis with small abscesses

- Round or oval copper-colored organisms with thick walls and septation (so-called "Medlar bodies," sclerotic bodies, or copper pennies). Spores within giant cells and extracellularly are visible even without special stains
- Numerous plasma cells and eosinophils

DD: Phaeohyphomycosis (budding but no septation of hyphae); other deep fungal or mycobacterial infections, for example, tuberculosis cutis verrucosa or leprosy; tertiary syphilis; leishmaniasis; sporotrichosis; verrucous carcinoma.

Reference

Elgart, G. W. (1996). Chromoblastomycosis. *Dermatol Clin*, **14**(1), 77–83.

Lokuhetty, M. D., Alahakoon, V. S., Kularatne, B. D., & De Silva, M. V. (2007). Ziehl-Neelsen and Wade-Fite stains to demonstrate medlar bodies of chromoblastomycosis. *J Cutan Pathol*, **34**(1), 71–72.

Minotto, R., Albano Edelweiss, M. I., & Scroferneker, M. L. (2017). Study on the organization of cellular elements in the granulomatous lesion caused by chromoblastomycosis. *J Cutan Pathol*, **44**(11), 915–918.

Skupsky, H., & Junkins-Hopkins, J. (2017). Counterfeit pennies: Distinguishing chromoblastomycosis from phaeohyphomycotic infections. *Am J Dermatopathol*, **39**(6), 485–487.

2.3 Systemic Mycoses (Deep Fungal Infections)

Systemic dissemination of fungal infections usually occurs via primary pulmonary infection, mostly in immunocompromised patients. Conversely, primary cutaneous fungal infection with subsequent dissemination is the exception.

Reference

Abbott, J. J., Hamacher, K. L., & Ahmed, I. (2006). In situ hybridization in cutaneous deep fungal infections: A valuable diagnostic adjunct to fungal morphology and tissue cultures. *J Cutan Pathol*, **33**(6), 426–432.

Fernandez-Flores, A., Saeb-Lima, M., & Arenas-Guzman, R. (2014). Morphological findings of deep cutaneous fungal infections. *Am J Dermatopathol*, **36**(7), 531–553.

Kauffman, C. A. (2006). Endemic mycoses: Blastomycosis, histoplasmosis, and sporotrichosis. *Infect Dis Clin North Am*, **20**(3), 645–662.

Lupi, O., Tyring, S. K., & McGinnis, M. R. (2005). Tropical dermatology: Fungal tropical diseases. *J Am Acad Dermatol*, **53**(6), 931–951.

Wiley, E. L., Beck, B., & Freeman, R. G. (1991). Reactivity of fungal organisms in tissue sections using anti-mycobacteria antibodies. *J Cutan Pathol*, **18**(3), 204–209.

2.3.1 Cryptococcosis (Torulosis, European Blastomycosis)

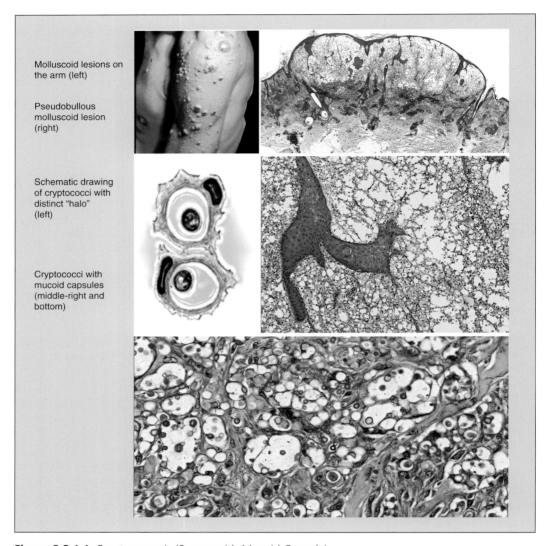

Molluscoid lesions on the arm (left)

Pseudobullous molluscoid lesion (right)

Schematic drawing of cryptococci with distinct "halo" (left)

Cryptococci with mucoid capsules (middle-right and bottom)

Figure 2.3.1.1 Cryptococcosis (Spores with Mucoid Capsule).

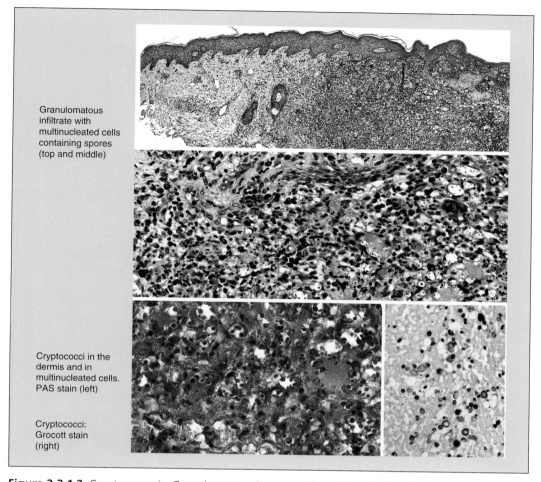

Granulomatous infiltrate with multinucleated cells containing spores (top and middle)

Cryptococci in the dermis and in multinucleated cells. PAS stain (left)

Cryptococci: Grocott stain (right)

Figure 2.3.1.2 Cryptococcosis, Granulomatous (Spores without Mucoid Capsules).

Cryptococcus spp. is a spherical opportunistic yeast and comprises various serotypes (A-D). *Cryptococcus neoformans and C. gattii,* which preferentially thrive in soil contaminated with the droppings of pigeons, may cause acute infections preferentially in immunocompromised patients. Primary cutaneous disease is rare; cutaneous symptoms are nonspecific. Remarkably, the infection is often overlooked, and patients often are not aware that they have cryptococcosis.

CF: Primary cutaneous infection by *Cryptococcus* spp. is rare. Infections usually start with pulmonary or CNS involvement, followed by hematogenous spreading. Concomitant cutaneous symptoms may present as acneiform papules, pustules, plaques, or umbilicated nodules resembling molluscum contagiosum, abscesses, or ulcerations without specific causes.

HF:

- Characteristic yeast surrounded by a wide clear mucoid capsule (Alcian blue and mucin stains are strikingly positive)
- Spores without gelatinous capsules may be present in large numbers, mostly within a mixed granulomatous infiltrate containing many multinucleated giant cells
- Often, exclusively intracytoplasmic spores (multinucleate giant cells) without capsule

DD: Blastomycosis; histoplasmosis; lobomycosis; molluscum; creeping skin lesions.

Reference

Chayakulkeeree, M., & Perfect, J. R. (2006). Cryptococcosis. *Infect Dis Clin North Am*, **20**(3), 507–544, v–vi.

Dimino-Emme, L., & Gurevitch, A. W. (1995). Cutaneous manifestations of disseminated cryptococcosis. *J Am Acad Dermatol*, **32**(5 Pt 2), 844–850.

Ramdial, P. K., Calonje, E., Sing, Y., Chotey, N. A., & Aboobaker, J. (2008). Molluscum-like cutaneous cryptococcosis: A histopathological and pathogenetic appraisal. *J Cutan Pathol*, **35**(11), 1007–1013.

Walsh, T. L., Bhanot, N., Murillo, M. A., Uchin, J. M., & Min, Z. (2017). Creeping skin lesions: Primary cutaneous cryptococcosis. *Am J Med*, **130**(6), 666–668.

2.3.2 North American Blastomycosis (Blastomycosis, Chicago Disease)

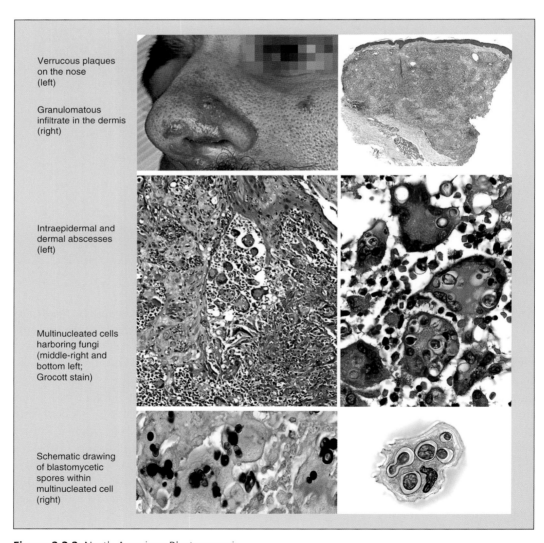

Verrucous plaques on the nose (left)

Granulomatous infiltrate in the dermis (right)

Intraepidermal and dermal abscesses (left)

Multinucleated cells harboring fungi (middle-right and bottom left; Grocott stain)

Schematic drawing of blastomycetic spores within multinucleated cell (right)

Figure 2.3.2 North American Blastomycosis.

Blastomyces dermatitidis, the causative organism of North American Blastomycosis, is a dimorphic fungus that affects humans and animals. Blastomycosis is a systemic disease and usually starts with pulmonary infection via inhalation of spores that are present in moist soil or rotten wood. Hematogenous dissemination leads to infection of the skin and other organs. Primary cutaneous blastomycosis with characteristic sporotrichoid spreading is very rare and may also occur in immunocompetent healthy persons. *Paracoccidioides brasiliensis* and *Cryptococcus neoformans* are responsible for the South American and the European forms of blastomycosis, respectively.

CF: The preferential site is the face. Slowly spreading verrucous papules or plaques, showing pustules and crusts, occasionally with raised borders and central regression and necrosis are typical.

HF:

- Dense inflammatory infiltrate in the dermis
- Intraepidermal and dermal neutrophilic
- Microabscesses, reminiscent of pemphigus vegetans or iododerma
- Granulomatous infiltrate with giant cells in the dermis
- Necrosis
- Double-contoured (refractile double wall) thick budding organisms (PAS or Gomori silver stain), extracellularly in the necrotic center, and within giant cells

DD: Pyoderma gangrenosum; tuberculosis; coccidioidomycosis; chromoblastosis; Sweet syndrome.

Reference

Azar, M. M., Relich, R. F., Schmitt, B. H., Spech, R. W., & Hage, C. A. (2014). Cutaneous blastomycosis masquerading as pyoderma gangrenosum. *J Clin Microbiol*, **52**(4), 1298–1300.

Ladizinski, B., & Piette, W. (2018). Disseminated cutaneous blastomycosis. *N Engl J Med*, **379**(1), 74.

Ouchi, T., Tamura, M., Nishimoto, S., Sato, T., & Ishiko, A. (2011). A case of blastomycosis-like pyoderma caused by mixed infection of Staphylococcus epidermidis and Trichophyton rubrum. *Am J Dermatopathol*, **33**(4), 397–399.

Wilkerson, A., King, R., Googe, P. B., Page, R. N., & Fulk, C. S. (2003). Sweet's syndrome-like blastomycosis. *Am J Dermatopathol*, **25**(2), 152–154.

2.3.3 Lobomycosis (Lobo Disease, Keloidal Blastomycosis, Blastomycoid Granuloma)

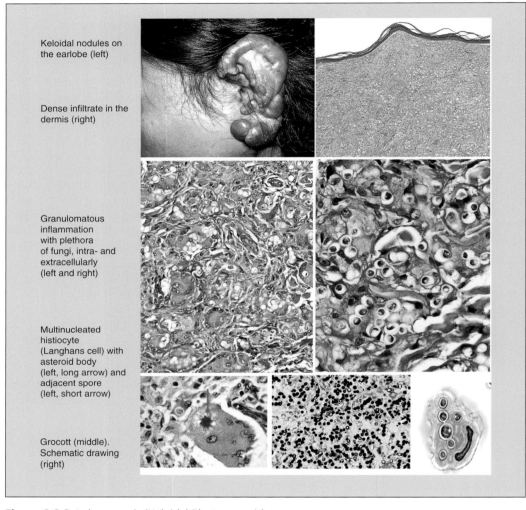

Keloidal nodules on the earlobe (left)

Dense infiltrate in the dermis (right)

Granulomatous inflammation with plethora of fungi, intra- and extracellularly (left and right)

Multinucleated histiocyte (Langhans cell) with asteroid body (left, long arrow) and adjacent spore (left, short arrow)

Grocott (middle). Schematic drawing (right)

Figure 2.3.3 Lobomycosis (Keloidal Blastomycosis).

CF: This variant of blastomycosis, caused by *Lacazia loboi* and discovered by the Brazilian dermatologist Jorge Lobo, is a chronic granulomatous disease of the skin and the subcutaneous tissue, producing nodular and keloidal lesions on the face, ears, and the limbs but also on any other site of the skin. Infections commonly occur in South and Central America. Typical are smooth-surfaced nodules resembling scars or keloids. Exophytic, cauliflower-like lesions are not unusual.

HF:

- Granulomatous inflammation in the dermis
- Diffuse proliferation of fungi
- Fungi between and within histiocytes and Langhans cells

DD: Blastomycosis; keloid.

Reference

Cabrera-Salom, C., Gonzalez, L. F., Rolon, M., & Sanchez, B. F. (2017). Keloids on the ears. *Int J Dermatol*, **56**(8), 819–821.

Fuchs, J., Milbradt, R., & Pecher, S. A. (1990). Lobomycosis (keloidal blastomycosis): Case reports and overview. *Cutis*, **46**(3), 227–234.

2.3.4 Histoplasmosis

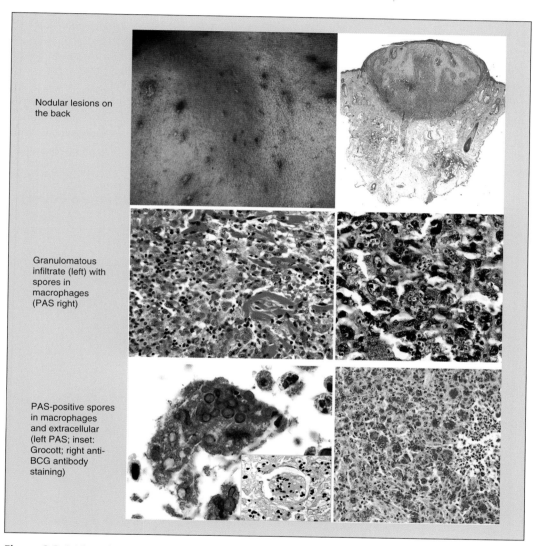

Nodular lesions on the back

Granulomatous infiltrate (left) with spores in macrophages (PAS right)

PAS-positive spores in macrophages and extracellular (left PAS; inset: Grocott; right anti-BCG antibody staining)

Figure 2.3.4 Histoplasmosis.

The dimorphic fungus *Histoplasma capsulatum* thrives in soil contaminated with bats' or birds' droppings. Primary pulmonary infection occurs via inhalation of spores, often followed by hematogenous spread to other organs. Children and immunocompromised patients are at an increased risk of infection.

CF: Primary cutaneous histoplasmosis that is caused by local infection is extremely rare and may present with a characteristic chancriform ulcer. In general, hematogenous dissemination of *Histoplasma capsulatum* to the skin shows a plethora of different clinical lesions: mostly multiform erythema, erythema nodosum, panniculitis, papules, nodules, or small ulcers.

HF:

- Lymphohistiocytic infiltrate with plasma cells (early) or granulomatous infiltrate (late)
- Small non-capsulated spores (PAS-positive) mostly in macrophages
- Leukocytic vasculitis may be present
- Prominent parasitization of epidermal keratinocytes has been observed

DD: Leishmaniasis (showing PAS-negative amastigotes); cryptococcosis; granuloma inguinale; erythema nodosum.

Reference

Honarpisheh, H. H., Curry, J. L., Richards, K., Nagarajan, P., Aung, P. P., Torres-Cabala, C. A., . . . Tetzlaff, M. T. (2016). Cutaneous histoplasmosis with prominent parasitization of epidermal keratinocytes: Report of a case. *J Cutan Pathol*, **43**(12), 1155–1160.

Medeiros, A. A., Marty, S. D., Tosh, F. E., & Chin, T. D. (1966). Erythema nodosum and erythema multiforme as clinical manifestations of histoplasmosis in a community outbreak. *N Engl J Med*, **274**(8), 415–420.

Ollague Sierra, J. E., & Ollague Torres, J. M. (2013). New clinical and histological patterns of acute disseminated histoplasmosis in human immunodeficiency virus-positive patients with acquired immunodeficiency syndrome. *Am J Dermatopathol*, **35**(2), 205–212.

2.3.5 Coccidioidomycosis (Desert or Valley Fever, San Joaquin Fever)

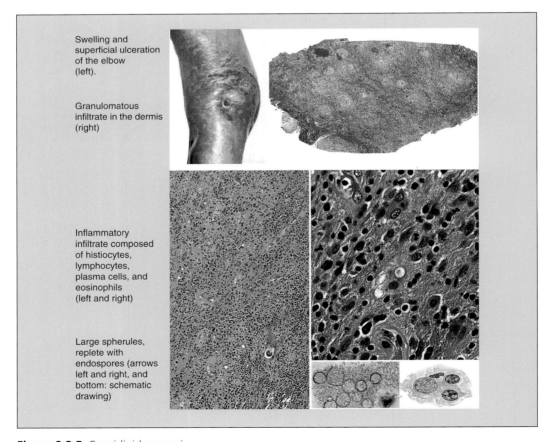

Swelling and superficial ulceration of the elbow (left).

Granulomatous infiltrate in the dermis (right)

Inflammatory infiltrate composed of histiocytes, lymphocytes, plasma cells, and eosinophils (left and right)

Large spherules, replete with endospores (arrows left and right, and bottom: schematic drawing)

Figure 2.3.5 Coccidioidomycosis.

CF: Pulmonary infection with the highly infective and ubiquitous soil fungus *Coccidioides immitis* or the closely related *Coccidioides posadasii*. Coccidioidomycosis is a potentially fatal disease. Dissemination is rare and usually involves the bone and CNS. Cutaneous lesions may present as erythema nodosum, diffuse maculopapular exanthem, erythema multiforme, papules, and nodules. Verrucous lesions, ulcers, and deep abscesses with draining sinus tracts are not uncommon.

HF: Granulomatous inflammation, containing large spherules, containing endospores.
DD: Erythema nodosum; arthritis; bursitis.

Reference

Carpenter, J. B., Feldman, J. S., Leyva, W. H., & DiCaudo, D. J. (2010). Clinical and pathologic characteristics of disseminated cutaneous coccidioidomycosis. *J Am Acad Dermatol*, **62**(5), 831–837.

DiCaudo, D. J. (2006). Coccidioidomycosis: A review and update. *J Am Acad Dermatol*, **55**(6), 929–942.

2.3.6 Paracoccidioidomycosis (South American Blastomycosis)

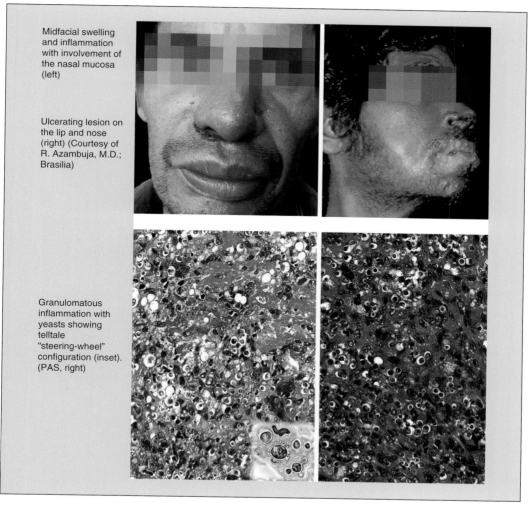

Midfacial swelling and inflammation with involvement of the nasal mucosa (left)

Ulcerating lesion on the lip and nose (right) (Courtesy of R. Azambuja, M.D.; Brasilia)

Granulomatous inflammation with yeasts showing telltale "steering-wheel" configuration (inset). (PAS, right)

Figure 2.3.6 Paracoccidioidomycosis.

This deep mycotic disease is caused by inhalation of *Paracoccidioides brasiliensis*. Paracoccidioidomycosis is endemic in South and Central America.

CF: The acute pulmonary infection may resemble pneumonia. Hepatosplenomegaly and bone marrow dysfunction are other systemic symptoms of the potentially fatal infection, particularly in young patients. Cutaneous facial lesions are common, around the nose and the mouth, often in conjunction with painful, slowly expanding, hyperkeratotic mucosal ulcerations.

HF: Plasma cell-rich granulomatous infiltrate, mostly under a hyperkeratotic epidermis, with pseudoepitheliomatous hyperplasia in the dermis. PAS-positive yeasts show a typical steering-wheel pattern with multiple narrow-spaced tiny buds radiating peripherally from the round to oval center of the spore.

DD: Other deep fungal infections.

Reference

Catano, J. C., & Morales, M. (2015). Cutaneous paracoccidioidomycosis. *Am J Trop Med Hyg*, **93**(3), 433–434.

Garcia Bustinduy, M., Guimera, F. J., Arevalo, P., Castro, C., Saez, M., Dorta Alom, S., . . . Garcia Montelongo, R. (2000). Cutaneous primary paracoccidioidomycosis. *J Eur Acad Dermatol Venereol*, **14**(2), 113–117.

2.3.7 Emmonsiosis

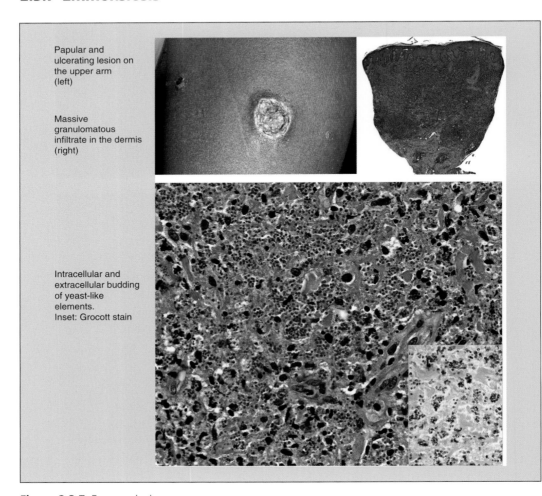

Papular and ulcerating lesion on the upper arm (left)

Massive granulomatous infiltrate in the dermis (right)

Intracellular and extracellular budding of yeast-like elements.
Inset: Grocott stain

Figure 2.3.7 Emmonsiosis.

Emmonsia, a dimorphic fungus with phylogenetic relationship to *Blastomyces*. *Emmonsia* comprises various species, including *Emmonsia pasteuriana*, which may be pathogenic to humans, especially in advanced HIV disease. Pulmonary involvement is frequent. Clinically, histopathologically, and radiologically, emmonsiosis masquerades as histoplasmosis.

CF: Erythematous plaques and papules with central umbilication, necrosis, and ulceration.

HF: Chronic inflammation with granuloma formation. Intracellular and extracellular budding of yeast-like elements are seen in over 90% of biopsies. Organisms highlighted by PAS, Grocott methenamine silver stain (GMS), or by *Histoplasma* antigen (cross-reactivity with *Emmonsia* spp.). Confirmation of the diagnosis should be based on fungal culture or sequence molecular analysis.

DD: Other deep fungal infections; histoplasmosis; sporotrichosis; blastomycosis; varicella; Kaposi sarcoma; drug reaction.

Reference

Feng, P., Yin, S., Zhu, G., Li, M., Wu, B., Xie, Y., . . . Lai, W. (2015). Disseminated infection caused by Emmonsia pasteuriana in a renal transplant recipient. *J Dermatol*, **42**(12), 1179–1182.

Kenyon, C., Bonorchis, K., Corcoran, C., Meintjes, G., Locketz, M., Lehloenya, R., . . . Govender, N. P. (2013). A dimorphic fungus causing disseminated infection in South Africa. *N Engl J Med*, **369**(15), 1416–1424.

Malik, R., Capoor, M. R., Vanidassane, I., Gogna, A., Singh, A., Sen, B., . . . Chakrabarti, A. (2016). Disseminated Emmonsia pasteuriana infection in India: A case report and a review. *Mycoses*, **59**(2), 127–132. doi:10.1111/myc.12437

Schwartz, I. S., Govender, N. P., Corcoran, C., Dlamini, S., Prozesky, H., Burton, R., . . . Kenyon, C. (2015). Clinical characteristics, diagnosis, management, and outcomes of disseminated Emmonsiosis: A retrospective case series. *Clin Infect Dis*, **61**(6), 1004–1012.

2.4 Opportunistic Fungal Infections

2.4.1 Aspergillosis (Alternaria)

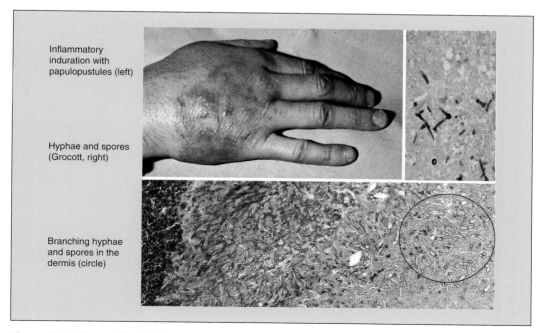

Inflammatory induration with papulopustules (left)

Hyphae and spores (Grocott, right)

Branching hyphae and spores in the dermis (circle)

Figure 2.4.1 Aspergillosis (Alternaria).

Aspergillosis is an infection by the opportunistic fungus *Aspergillus fumigatus* or other *Aspergillus species* (*A. niger, A. flavus*), which are ubiquitously found in air, soil, and decaying organic matter. Immunocompromised patients carry an increased risk of infection.

CF: Primary pulmonary infection, rarely with pulmonary fungal ball (aspergilloma) in a preexisting lung cavity. Disseminated disease with cutaneous fungal emboli showing black cutaneous eschars and infarcts, often evolving from banal superficial wounds in immunosuppressed patients.

HF:

- Aspergillus hyphae within vessel lumina, walls, and in adjacent dermis
- Hyphal septation with 45° dichotomous branching

- Associated thrombi
- GMS-, PAS-positive hyphae and spores
- Concomitant inflammatory reaction
- PCR for demonstration of *Aspergillus* spp. in the blood (fungemia)

DD: Mucormycosis   (Zygomycosis; Phycomycosis).

Reference

Goel, R., & Wallace, M. L. (2001). Pseudoepitheliomatous hyperplasia secondary to cutaneous aspergillus. *Am J Dermatopathol*, **23**(3), 224–226.

Shinohara, M. M., Miller, C. J., & Seykora, J. T. (2011). Pigmented fruiting bodies and birefringent crystals in a surgical wound: A clue to Aspergillus niger infection. *J Cutan Pathol*, **38**(8), 603–606.

2.4.2 Zygomycosis (Mucormycosis; Phycomycosis)

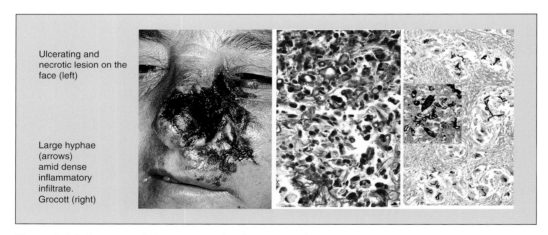

Figure 2.4.2 Zygomycosis (Mucormycosis; Phycomycosis).

The ubiquitous saprophytic organisms of the *Mucor* spp., *Rhizomucor, Rhizopus,* and *Cunninghamella* are found in soil and in decaying organic material but rarely cause disease.

CF: Diabetic and immunocompromised patients are at risk of developing infection, in particular, of the nasal cavity and sinuses, which may be followed by systemic spread to the brain and the respiratory system. Facial edema, orbital cellulitis, nasal discharge, and cavernous sinus thrombosis are common findings in acute infections.

HF:

- Large hyphae branching at right angles
- Lack of septa
- Fungi invade vessel walls and show intravascular growth
- Inflammatory reaction may vary

DD: Aspergillosis (hyphae with typical septa and not branching at right angles); granulomatous pyoderma.

Reference

Geller, J. D., Peters, M. S., & Su, W. P. (1993). Cutaneous mucormycosis resembling superficial granulomatous pyoderma in an immunocompetent host. *J Am Acad Dermatol, 29*(3), 462–465.

Requena, L., Sitthinamsuwan, P., Santonja, C., Fernandez-Figueras, M. T., Rodriguez-Peralto, J. L., Argenyi, Z., . . . Kutzner, H. (2012). Cutaneous and mucosal mucormycosis mimicking pancreatic panniculitis and gouty panniculitis. *J Am Acad Dermatol, 66*(6), 975–984.

Umbert, I. J., & Su, W. P. (1989). Cutaneous mucormycosis. *J Am Acad Dermatol, 21*(6), 1232–1234.

2.4.3 Hyalohyphomycosis

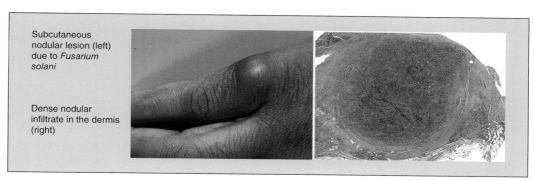

Subcutaneous nodular lesion (left) due to *Fusarium solani*

Dense nodular infiltrate in the dermis (right)

Figure 2.4.3 Hyalohyphomycosis.

The relevant infectious organisms are *Fusarium* and *Pseudallescheria boydii* that are hyaline, colorless molds, ubiquitously present in soil. These molds are glassy (hyalo-), non-pigmented, and have septate hyphae.

CF: Superficial hemorrhagic and necrotic skin lesions, ecthyma gangrenosum-like flat ulcers, subcutaneous nodular and mycetoma-like infiltrates are found mostly in immunocompromised patients. Secondary infection of superficial wounds may occur.

HF: Inflamed nodules and eschars with ischemic necrosis, resulting from septic fungus-invasion into vessels. PAS-positive fungi.

DD: Other deep fungal infections; ecthyma gangrenosum; bacterial abscess; squamous cell carcinoma.

Reference

Arrese, J. E., Pierard-Franchimont, C., & Pierard, G. E. (1996). Fatal hyalohyphomycosis following Fusarium onychomycosis in an immunocompromised patient. *Am J Dermatopathol, 18*(2), 196–198.

Bushelman, S. J., Callen, J. P., Roth, D. N., & Cohen, L. M. (1995). Disseminated Fusarium solani infection. *J Am Acad Dermatol, 32*(2 Pt 2), 346–351.

Griffin, T. D., McFarland, J. P., & Johnson, W. C. (1991). Hyalohyphomycosis masquerading as squamous cell carcinoma. *J Cutan Pathol, 18*(2), 116–119.

2.4.4 Phaeohyphomycosis

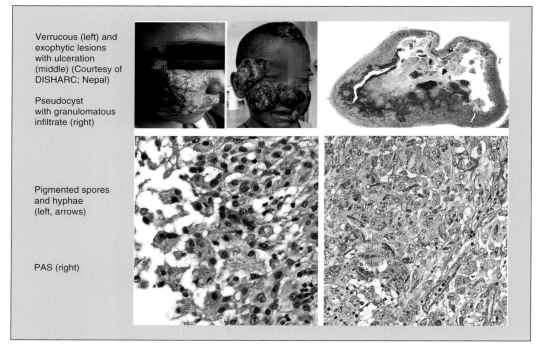

Verrucous (left) and exophytic lesions with ulceration (middle) (Courtesy of DISHARC; Nepal)

Pseudocyst with granulomatous infiltrate (right)

Pigmented spores and hyphae (left, arrows)

PAS (right)

Figure 2.4.4 Phaeohyphomycosis.

CF: The term *dematiaceous* denotes organisms, in particular fungi, which produce a dark pigment. This group of pathogenic organisms causes the fungal infections phaeohyphomycosis (phaeo- also meaning *pigmented*) and chromoblastomycosis, which may present with various clinical symptoms, ranging from superficial pigmented lesions as tinea nigra to subcutaneous nodules and fulminant abscess formation. Systemic dissemination via hematogenic spread in immunocompromised patients results in a severe life-threatening condition.

HF:

- Pseudocystic and dermal neutrophilic abscesses
- Granulomatous inflammation with plasma cells
- Abundant budding spores and branching pigmented hyphae
- Demonstration of melanin by Fontana-Masson stain

DD: Chromoblastomycosis; mycetomas.

Reference

Kapatia, G., Pandey, T., Kakkar, N., Kaur, H., & Verma, R. (2019). Facial phaeohyphomycosis in an immunocompetent individual: A rare presentation of a rare fungus. *Am J Dermatopathol*, **41**(2), 137–139.

Ronan, S. G., Uzoaru, I., Nadimpalli, V., Guitart, J., & Manaligod, J. R. (1993). Primary cutaneous phaeohyphomycosis: Report of seven cases. *J Cutan Pathol*, **20**(3), 223–228.

2.4.5 Protothecosis, Cutaneous

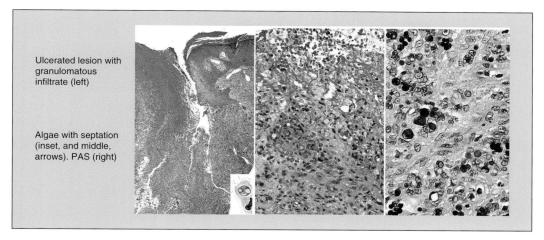

Ulcerated lesion with granulomatous infiltrate (left)

Algae with septation (inset, and middle, arrows). PAS (right)

Figure 2.4.5 Protothecosis, Cutaneous.

CF: *Prototheca wickerhamii* and *Prototheca zopfi*, achlorophyllic algae, are ubiquitous present in soil, plants, and contaminated water. When entering skin wounds in immuno-compromised patients, they may produce a nodular and ulcerating inflammation.

HF: Inflammatory reaction with necrotizing and caseating granuloma, containing algae extracellularly or within giant cells. Typically, the large, round organisms show internal septation with endospores.

DD: Granulomatous foreign body reactions; deep mycoses.

Reference

Hillesheim, P. B., & Bahrami, S. (2011). Cutaneous protothecosis. *Arch Pathol Lab Med*, **135**(7), 941–944.

Walsh, S. V., Johnson, R. A., & Tahan, S. R. (1998). Prototothecosis: An unusual cause of chronic subcutaneous and soft tissue infection. *Am J Dermatopathol*, **20**(4), 379–382.

CHAPTER 3

Viral Infections

CHAPTER MENU

3.1 Herpes Viruses
   3.1.1 Herpes Simplex (HSV-1, HSV-2)
   3.1.2 Varizella/Zoster Virus (VZV/HHV-3)
   3.1.3 Burkitt Lymphoma; Epstein-Barr Virus (HHV-4 EBV)
   3.1.4 Hairy Leukoplakia HHV-4; Epstein-Barr Virus; EBV)
   3.1.5 Cytomegalovirus (CMV; HHV-5)
   3.1.6 Exanthema Subitum (HHV-6) (Roseola Infantum, 6th Disease)
   3.1.7 Pityriasis Rosea (HHV-7)
   3.1.8 AIDS-Kaposi Sarcoma (HHV-8)
   3.1.9 Multicentric Castleman's Disease (HHV-8)
3.2 Human Papilloma Virus (HPV)
   3.2.1 Verruca Vulgaris
   3.2.2 Variant: Verrucae Planae
   3.2.3 Variant: Condylomata Acuminata
   3.2.4 Differential Diagnosis: Acrokeratosis Verruciformis (Hopf)
   3.2.5 Bowenoid Papulosis
   3.2.6 Epidermodysplasia Verruciformis (Lewandowsky–Lutz); Verrucosis Generalisata
3.3 Viral Exanthema
   3.3.1 Measles

3.4 Parvovirus Infections and Coxsackievirus Infections
   3.4.1 Erythema Infectiosum; (Slapped Cheek Disease; Fifth Disease)
   3.4.2 Papular Purpuric Gloves-and-Socks Syndrome
   3.4.3 Hand-Foot-and-Mouth Disease (Coxsackie Virus)
3.5 Polyoma Virus Infections
   3.5.1 Trichodysplasia Spinulosa
   3.5.2 Merkel Cell Carcinoma (Primary Neuroendocrine Carcinoma of the Skin; Trabecular Carcinoma of Toker)
3.6 Poxviruses
   3.6.1 Orthopox Virus Infections
   3.6.2 Parapox Virus Infections
3.7 Other Skin Diseases with Suspected Viral Association
   3.7.1 Asymmetric Periflexural Exanthema of Childhood
   3.7.2 Eruptive Pseudoangiomatosis
   3.7.3 Gianotti–Crosti Syndrome
   3.7.4 Pityriasis Lichenoides

°no pictures

Atlas of Clinical Dermatopathology: Infectious and Parasitic Dermatoses, First Edition. Günter Burg,
Heinz Kutzner, Werner Kempf, Josef Feit, and Omar Sangueza.
© 2021 John Wiley & Sons Ltd. Published 2021 by John Wiley & Sons Ltd.

Viruses (DNA and RNA) are obligate intracellular parasites. Their replication depends on the metabolism of the host cells. Viruses, due to their tropisms for different tissues (epithelia, endothelia, nervous system, vascular structures), cause a plethora of clinical cutaneous symptoms, reaching from inconspicuous exanthemas to papules, vesicles, and necrotic lesions. These morphological patterns allow for a more practical and clinical approach toward differentiation of the various viral dermatoses than the taxonomy of viruses.

3.1 Herpes Viruses

3.1.1 Herpes Simplex (HSV-1, HSV-2)

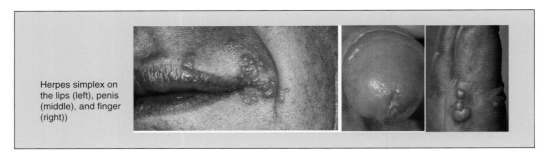

Herpes simplex on the lips (left), penis (middle), and finger (right))

Figure 3.1.1 Herpes Simplex.

The clinically relevant human herpes virus (HHV) family comprises eight types of herpes virus. Herpes simplex virus type 1 and 2 (HSV-1, HSV-2) are the most common ones. HSV-1 and 2 together with varicella zoster virus (VZV/HHV-3) belong to the α-subfamily of human herpes viruses. Primary infection in children may be subclinical in most cases, or presents as herpetic gingivostomatitis, sometimes with severe symptoms (Aphthoid Pospischill–Feyrter). In a minority of adults, recurrent labial or genital herpes simplex may appear, following reactivation by various external or internal stimuli.

CF: Pathognomonic indicators are burning and itching sensations followed by the eruption of grouped tense vesicles with erythema, preferentially on the lips (HSV type 1) or the genital mucosa (HSV type 2). Rapid erosion of vesicles is followed by crust formation. Chronic ulcerative lesions are seen in immunocompromised individuals. Secondary inoculation of primary eczematous (atopic) dermatosis with herpes viruses results in widespread skin involvement (eczema herpeticatum; Kaposi's varicelliform eruption).

HF: The histopathologic changes in herpes simplex and in varizella/zoster eruptions are basically the same. Differentiation can be achieved by immunohistochemistry or PCR.

- Inter- and intracellular edema of the epidermis
- Intraepidermal acantholytic blister formation
- Epidermis:
  - Ballooning degeneration of keratinocytes
  - Necrotic keratinocytes with swollen pyknotic ("steel-gray") nuclei
  - Syncytial multinucleated epithelial giant cells (positive Tzanck smear)
- Dermal edema
- Predominantly lymphocytic, mixed cellular infiltrate in the dermis with many eosinophils
- Lymphocytic vasculitis

- Secondary leukocytoclastic vasculitis exclusively in VZV infection (this virus is both epitheliotropic and endotheliotropic)
- Concomitant cytomegalovirus infection may alter the histological features

DD: Other viral eruptions; drug eruption; acute graft-versus-host reaction; erythema multiforme; non-viral ulcers; pyoderma gangrenosum; Rickettsiosis.

Reference

Boyd, A. S., Zwerner, J. P., & Miller, J. L. (2012). Herpes simplex virus-induced plasmacytic atypia. *J Cutan Pathol*, **39**(2), 270–273.

Garib, G., Hughey, L. C., Elmets, C. A., Cafardi, J. A., & Andea, A. A. (2013). Atypical presentation of exophytic herpes simplex virus type 2 with concurrent cytomegalovirus infection: A significant pitfall in diagnosis. *Am J Dermatopathol*, **35**(3), 371–376.

Laggis, C., Wada, D., Shah, A., & Zussman, J. (2020). Eosinophils are surprisingly common in biopsy specimens of cutaneous herpes simplex virus and varicella zoster virus infections: Results of a comprehensive histopathologic and clinical appraisal. *J Cutan Pathol*, **47**(1), 6–11.

Pomerantz, H., Wang, H., Heilman, E. R., Sharon, V. R., & Gottesman, S. P. (2020). Peculiar vegetative tumor-like genital herpes simplex nodules with brisk tissue eosinophilia in patients with human immunodeficiency virus infection. *J Cutan Pathol*, **7**(2), 150–153.

Saunderson, R. B., Tng, V., Watson, A., & Scurry, J. (2016). Perianal herpes simplex virus infection misdiagnosed with pyoderma gangrenosum: Case of the month from the Case Consultation Committee of the International Society for the Study of Vulvovaginal Disease. *J Low Genit Tract Dis*, **20**(2), e14–15.

3.1.2 Varizella/Zoster Virus (VZV/HHV-3)

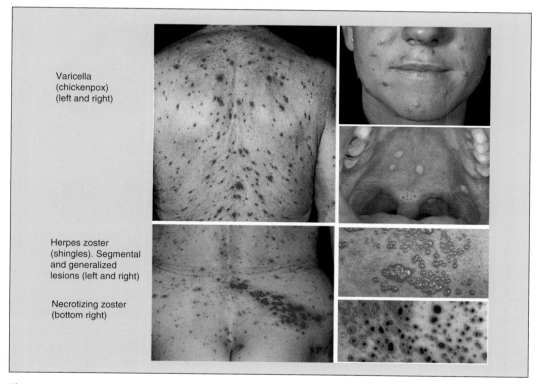

Varicella (chickenpox) (left and right)

Herpes zoster (shingles). Segmental and generalized lesions (left and right)

Necrotizing zoster (bottom right)

Figure 3.1.2 Varicella/Zoster.

The VZV/HHV-3 virus infection surfaces under different clinical morphologies, depending on the age and the immune status of the patient: while the initial VZV contact in children causes varicella (chickenpox), secondary virus reactivation in the elderly or in immunocompromised individuals, in particular in HIV/AIDS patients, manifests as herpes zoster.

3.1.2.1 Varicella (Chickenpox)

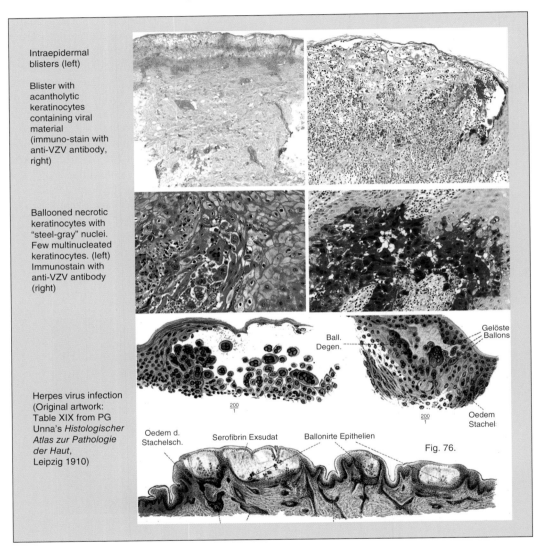

Intraepidermal blisters (left)

Blister with acantholytic keratinocytes containing viral material (immuno-stain with anti-VZV antibody, right)

Ballooned necrotic keratinocytes with "steel-gray" nuclei. Few multinucleated keratinocytes. (left) Immunostain with anti-VZV antibody (right)

Herpes virus infection (Original artwork: Table XIX from PG Unna's *Histologischer Atlas zur Pathologie der Haut*, Leipzig 1910)

Ball. Degen.
Gelöste Ballons
Oedem Stachel
Oedem d. Stachelsch.
Serofibrin Exsudat
Ballonirte Epithelien
Fig. 76.

Figure 3.1.2.1 Herpes Simplex; Varicella (Chickenpox)/Zoster (Shingles).

CF: Highly contagious viral disease, which primarily affects the respiratory tract and then spreads hematogenously, producing a characteristic polymorphic papulovesicular eruption, involving almost all parts of the integument as well as the palate, but characteristically sparing the palms and soles. Cutaneous lesions usually are in different stages of evolution, showing early lesions and older necrotizing lesions with crust formation side by side (the so-called metachronous synchrony of cutaneous lesions).

HF: The histopathological pattern is identical with herpes simplex infections, albeit with the production of rather large flaccid acantholytic vesicles.

DD: Generalized zoster; other vesicular or pustular dermatoses; psoriasis pustulosa; smallpox; monkey pox (which may look identical both clinically and histopathologically; endemic to Central Africa/Democratic Republic of Congo).

Reference

Burgard, B., Smola, S., Vogt, T., & Muller, C. S. L. (2018). Small vessel vasculitis in herpes zoster-discussion of current aspects of varicella zoster virus vasculopathy. *Am J Dermatopathol*, **40**(8), 602–604.

King, D. F., & King, L. A. (1986). Giant cells in lesions of varicella and herpes zoster. *Am J Dermatopathol*, **8**(5), 456–458.

McDonald, H. H., Corsini, L. M., Siddiqui, H. A., & Kowalewski, C. (2018). Granulomatous reaction after complete resolution of primary varicella. *Am J Dermatopathol*, **40**(1), 49–51.

Porto, D. A., Comfere, N. I., Myers, L. M., & Abbott, J. J. (2010). Pseudolymphomatous reaction to varicella zoster virus vaccination: Role of viral in situ hybridization. *J Cutan Pathol*, **37**(10), 1098–1102.

3.1.2.2 Herpes Zoster (Shingles)

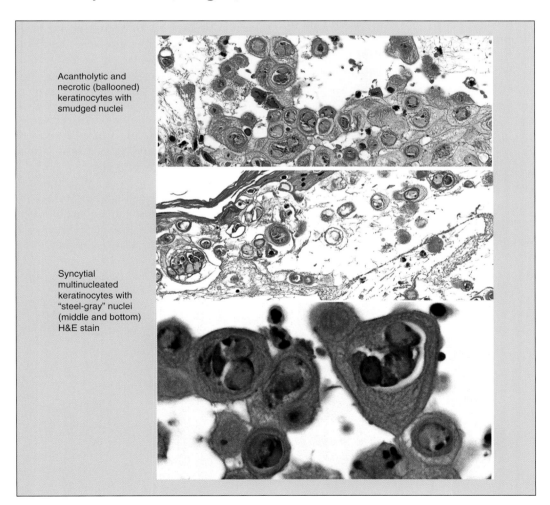

Acantholytic and necrotic (ballooned) keratinocytes with smudged nuclei

Syncytial multinucleated keratinocytes with "steel-gray" nuclei (middle and bottom) H&E stain

Figure 3.1.2.2.1 Herpes Simplex; Varicella (Chickenpox)/Zoster (Shingles).

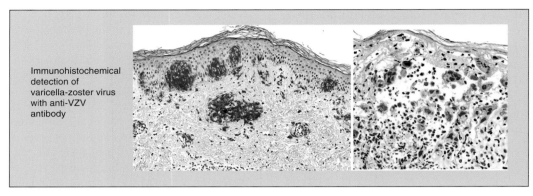

Immunohistochemical detection of varicella-zoster virus with anti-VZV antibody

Figure 3.1.2.2.2 Varicella (Chickenpox)/Zoster (Shingles).

Complete or partial loss of immune protection against varicella/zoster virus in conjunction with various external or internal factors leads to reactivation of the "dormant" virus (latent infection with virus within the ganglions of nerves) and to the development of mostly unilateral dermatomal cutaneous lesions. Rare "ectopic" and generalized eruptions occur via hematogenous spread.

CF: Painful segmental unilateral or generalized eruption of papulovesicles, which may be hemorrhagic and become pustular.

HF: Histology is the same as in herpes simplex or varicella. Remarkably, herpes zoster may go along with leukocytoclastic vasculitis and vasculopathic changes, often remote from the primary site of cutaneous infection.

DD: Varicella; zosteriform herpes simplex.

Reference

Boer, A., Herder, N., Blodorn-Schlicht, N., & Falk, T. (2006). Herpes incognito most commonly is herpes zoster and its histopathologic pattern is distinctive! *Am J Dermatopathol,* **28**(2), 181–186.

Burgard, B., Smola, S., Vogt, T., & Muller, C. S. L. (2018). Small vessel vasculitis in herpes zoster – discussion of current aspects of varicella zoster virus vasculopathy. *Am J Dermatopathol,* **40**(8), 602–604.

Ferenczi, K., Rosenberg, A. S., McCalmont, T. H., Kwon, E. J., Elenitsas, R., & Somach, S. C. (2015). Herpes zoster granulomatous dermatitis: Histopathologic findings in a case series. *J Cutan Pathol,* **42**(10), 739–745.

King, D. F., & King, L. A. (1986). Giant cells in lesions of varicella and herpes zoster. *Am J Dermatopathol,* **8**(5), 456–458.

3.1.2.3 Special Feature: Necrotizing (Herpes) Zoster Folliculitis

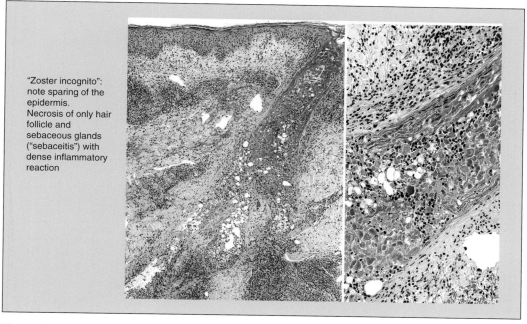

"Zoster incognito":
note sparing of the
epidermis.
Necrosis of only hair
follicle and
sebaceous glands
("sebaceitis") with
dense inflammatory
reaction

Figure 3.1.2.3 Special Feature: Necrotizing (Herpes) Zoster Folliculitis.

CF: Expanding widespread and painful papulonecrotic lesions, which may be confluent, eventually resolving with scars. Vesicles are usually lacking.

HF:

- Necrosis of only hair follicles and adnexal structures (sebaceous glands)
- Marked absence within the epidermis ("zoster incognito") of ballooning, acantholysis, blister formation, and multinucleated giant cells
- Accompanying dense dermal mixed inflammatory infiltrate, often resembling lymphoma or pseudolymphoma

- Immunohistochemical demonstration of virus within follicle epithelium

DD: Bacterial folliculitis.

Reference

Boer, A., Herder, N., Winter, K., & Falk, T. (2006). Herpes folliculitis: Clinical, histopathological, and molecular pathologic observations. *Br J Dermatol*, **154**(4), 743–746.

Nikkels, A. F., & Pierard, G. E. (2003). Necrotizing varicella zoster virus folliculitis. *Eur J Dermatol*, **13**(6), 587–589.

3.1.2.4 Special Feature: Zoster-Associated Vasculitis

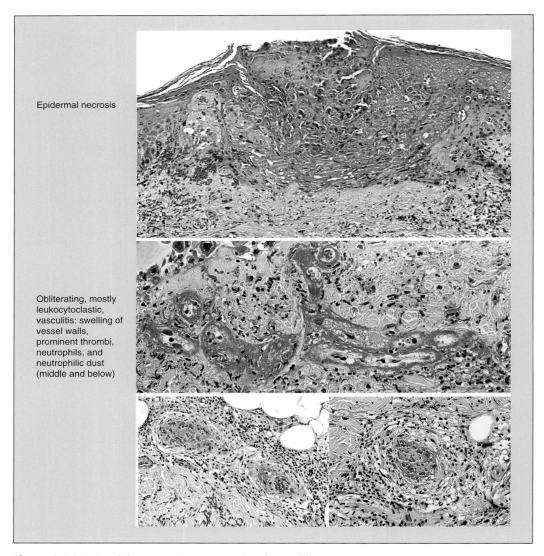

Epidermal necrosis

Obliterating, mostly leukocytoclastic, vasculitis: swelling of vessel walls, prominent thrombi, neutrophils, and neutrophilic dust (middle and below)

Figure 3.1.2.4 Special Feature: Zoster-Associated Vasculitis.

The VZV is both epitheliotropic and endotheliotropic, which explains the involvement of adjacent vessels in cutaneous VZV infection/herpes zoster. Lesions of herpes zoster may be hemorrhagic, and adjacent leukocytoclastic vasculitis is not unusual. Remarkably, concomitant vasculopathic changes may occur remotely from the site of the cutaneous infection, for example, in the brain or in internal organs. Synchronous involvement of both cutaneous sites and internal organs (e.g. liver) is not unusual in herpes zoster.

Reference

Burgard, B., Smola, S., Vogt, T., & Muller, C. S. L. (2018). Small vessel vasculitis in herpes zoster – discussion of current aspects of varicella zoster virus vasculopathy. *Am J Dermatopathol*, **40**(8), 602–604.

Clark, A. K., Dhossche, J., Korcheva, V. B., & Keller, J. J. (2018). Herpes zoster presenting as unilateral vasculitis. *Dermatol Online J*, **24**(11).

Gilden, D. H., Lipton, H. L., Wolf, J. S., Akenbrandt, W., Smith, J. E., Mahalingam, R., & Forghani, B. (2002). Two patients with unusual forms of varicella-zoster virus vasculopathy. *N Engl J Med*, **347**(19), 1500–1503.

Wollina, U., & Schonlebe, J. (2012). Segmental leukocytoclastic vasculitis in herpes zoster. *Int J Dermatol*, **51**(11), 1351–1352.

3.1.2.5 Postherpetic Cutaneous Reactions°

At sites of previous herpes zoster, various cutaneous reactions can occur:

- Granuloma annulare
- Sarcoidal granulomas
- Granulomatous folliculitis
- Granulomatous vasculitis
- Lichen planus
- Lichen sclerosus
- Pseudolymphoma
- Keloid

For further description and illustration, see Volume I on "Inflammatory Dermatoses."

Reference

Baalbaki, S. A., Malak, J. A., al-Khars, M. A., & Natarajan, S. (1994). Granulomatous vasculitis in herpes zoster scars. *Int J Dermatol*, **33**(4), 268–269.

3.1.3 Burkitt Lymphoma; Epstein-Barr Virus (HHV-4 EBV)

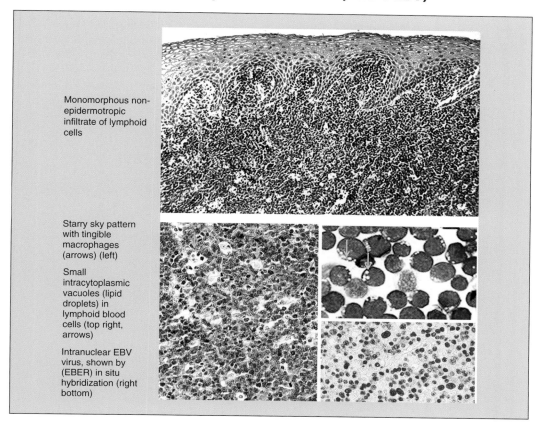

Monomorphous non-epidermotropic infiltrate of lymphoid cells

Starry sky pattern with tingible macrophages (arrows) (left)

Small intracytoplasmic vacuoles (lipid droplets) in lymphoid blood cells (top right, arrows)

Intranuclear EBV virus, shown by (EBER) in situ hybridization (right bottom)

Figure 3.1.3 Burkitt Lymphoma (HHV-4; Epstein-Barr Virus; EBV).
Source: Burg et al. (2019). *Atlas of Dermatopathology: Tumors, Nevi, and Cysts* (p. 459). Oxford: Wiley.

Burkitt lymphoma is a highly aggressive B-cell lymphoma, associated with Epstein-Barr virus/HHV-4 infection, featuring t(8;14) translocation with rearrangement of the *myc*-gene. HIV-induced immunodeficiency or malaria may be a predisposing factor.

CF: In equatorial Africa, Burkitt lymphoma preferentially involves the jaws of children. Outside of Africa, Burkitt lymphoma sporadically surfaces in children and in young adults. Immunocompromised patients (HIV/AIDS) are at particular risk of developing Burkitt lymphoma. The skin most commonly is affected by secondary invasion via regional lymph nodes.

HF:

- Diffuse cohesive monomorphous round cell infiltrate, lacking epidermotropism
- Medium-sized lymphoid cells with large nuclei and narrow basophilic cytoplasmatic rim showing small intracytoplasmic lipid vacuoles (adipophilin positive)
- Many mitotic figures and apoptotic cells
- Scattered pale macrophages (with distinct starry sky pattern), containing ingested remnants of apoptotic tumor cells

DD: Other B-cell lymphomas and pseudolymphomas; T-cell rich B-cell lymphoma; lymphocyte-rich Hodgkin lymphoma.

Reference

Burkitt, D. (1958). A sarcoma involving the jaws in African children. *Br J Surg*, **46**(197), 218–223.

Jacobson, M. A., Hutcheson, A. C., Hurray, D. H., Metcalf, J. S., & Thiers, B. H. (2006). Cutaneous involvement by Burkitt lymphoma. *J Am Acad Dermatol*, **54**(6), 1111–1113.

Mann, R. B., Jaffe, E. S., Braylan, R. C., Nanba, K., Frank, M. M., Ziegler, J. L., & Berard, C. W. (1976). Non-endemic Burkitts's lymphoma. A B-cell tumor related to germinal centers. *N Engl J Med*, **295**(13), 685–691.

Pettey, A. A., & Walsh, J. S. (2007). Cutaneous involvement with Burkitt-like lymphoma. *Am J Dermatopathol*, **29**(2), 184–186.

Rogge, T. (1975). [Burkitt's lymphoma with skin infiltrates]. *Hautarzt*, **26**(7), 379–382.

Rogers, A., Graves, M., Toscano, M., & Davis, L. (2014). A unique cutaneous presentation of Burkitt lymphoma. *Am J Dermatopathol*, **36**(12), 997–1001.

3.1.4 Hairy Leukoplakia (HHV-4; Epstein-Barr Virus; EBV)

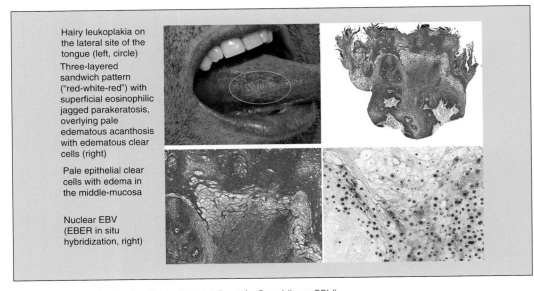

Hairy leukoplakia on the lateral site of the tongue (left, circle)

Three-layered sandwich pattern ("red-white-red") with superficial eosinophilic jagged parakeratosis, overlying pale edematous acanthosis with edematous clear cells (right)

Pale epithelial clear cells with edema in the middle-mucosa

Nuclear EBV (EBER in situ hybridization, right)

Figure 3.1.4 Hairy Leukoplakia (HHV-4 Epstein-Barr Virus; EBV).

CF: Distinct whitish hyperkeratosis ("lateral leukoplakia"), usually on the lateral side of the tongue, mostly in immunocompromised patients.

HF:

- Verrucous acanthosis and papillomatosis with superficial clefting
- Marked layering (red-white-red) of the mucosal epithelium
- Central "white" parts of epithelium showing epithelial clear cells with swollen, edematous cytoplasm and with prominent nuclei ("fish eye" cells)

DD: Precancerous leukoplakia; candida infection.

Reference

Fernandez, J. F., Benito, M. A., Lizaldez, E. B., & Montanes, M. A. (1990). Oral hairy leukoplakia: A histopathologic study of 32 cases. *Am J Dermatopathol*, **12**(6), 571–578.

Sandvej, K., Krenacs, L., Hamilton-Dutoit, S. J., Rindum, J. L., Pindborg, J. J., & Pallesen, G. (1992). Epstein-Barr virus latent and replicative gene expression in oral hairy leukoplakia. *Histopathology*, **20**(5), 387–395.

Southam, J. C., Felix, D. H., Wray, D., & Cubie, H. A. (1991). Hairy leukoplakia – a histological study. *Histopathology*, **19**(1), 63–67.

Winzer, M., Gilliar, U., & Ackerman, A. B. (1988). Hairy lesions of the oral cavity. Clinical and histopathologic differentiation of hairy leukoplakia from hairy tongue. *Am J Dermatopathol*, **10**(2), 155–159.

3.1.5 Cytomegalovirus (CMV; HHV-5)

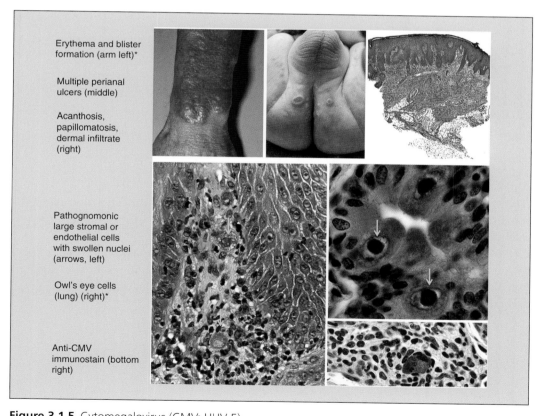

Figure 3.1.5 Cytomegalovirus (CMV; HHV-5).
*Source: Burg et al. (2015). *Atlas of Dermatopathology: Practical Differential Diagnosis by Clinicopathologic Pattern* (p. 90). Oxford: Wiley.

The infection starts with viremia, following primary oropharyngeal inoculation with the cytomegalovirus. Preferentially immunosuppressed and post-transplant patients are at risk of infection. Pathognomonic in the skin are small ulcers, but other clinical presentations of cytomegalovirus infection are not unusual.

CF: The skin is only rarely involved, showing small blisters with superficial ulceration and scale crust formation.

HF: A telltale sign are swollen and slightly detached endothelial cells with intracytoplasmic round basophilic inclusions ("owl's eye" cells). Rarely, these virus-laden cells may also be found in other tissue components (fibroblasts).

DD: Ecthyma contagiosum.

3.1.6 Exanthema Subitum (HHV-6) (Roseola Infantum, 6th Disease)

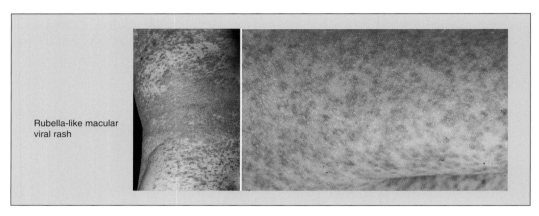

Rubella-like macular viral rash

Figure 3.1.6 Exanthema Subitum (HHV-6) (Roseola Infantum).

Almost all children show evidence of HHV-6 infection early in life. The virus remains in a latent state, but reactivation may occur.

CF: Sudden onset of high fever is followed by a transient rubella-like rapidly clearing macular exanthem, sparing the face with no enanthem.

HF:

- Superficial lymphocytic dermal infiltrate – similar to other viral and paraviral exanthems
- Sparse spongiosis with minimal exocytosis. Vasculitic changes are lacking

DD: Other viral exanthemas allergic drug reactions (rare).

3.1.7 Pityriasis Rosea (HHV-7)

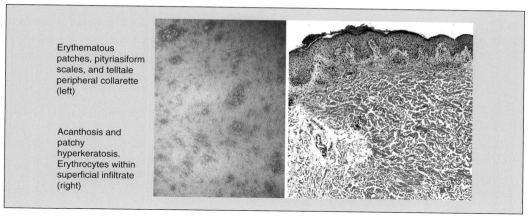

Erythematous patches, pityriasiform scales, and telltale peripheral collarette (left)

Acanthosis and patchy hyperkeratosis. Erythrocytes within superficial infiltrate (right)

Figure 3.1.7.1 Pityriasis Rosea (HHV-7).
Source: Burg et al. (2015). *Atlas of Dermatopathology: Practical Differential Diagnosis by Clinicopathologic Pattern* (p. 28). Oxford: Wiley.

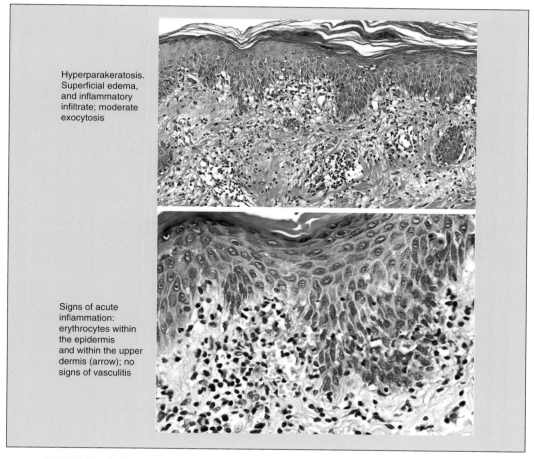

Hyperparakeratosis. Superficial edema, and inflammatory infiltrate; moderate exocytosis

Signs of acute inflammation: erythrocytes within the epidermis and within the upper dermis (arrow); no signs of vasculitis

Figure 3.1.7.2 Pityriasis Rosea (HHV-7).
Source: Burg et al. (2015). *Atlas of Dermatopathology: Practical Differential Diagnosis by Clinicopathologic Pattern* (p. 29). Oxford: Wiley.

A causative agent in pityriasis rosea, most likely the human herpes virus 7 HHV-7, is highly suggestive, but has not yet definitely been confirmed.

CF: Disseminated small erythematous patches with superficial peripheral scaling; incipient solitary oval herald patch (tâche mère) with prominent collarette.

HF: Corresponds to eczematous dermatitis

- Focal psoriasiform hyperparakeratosis (often with serum exudate)
- Slight spongiosis and exocytosis, sometimes with intraepidermal erythrocytes (acute stage)
- Patchy lymphocytic infiltrate in the upper dermis; remarkably, plasma cells are lacking

- Exocytosis of erythrocytes, but no vasculitic changes

DD: Other viral exanthema; secondary syphilis (with plasma cells!); tinea corporis; drug eruption; erythema multiforme.

Reference

Drago, F., Broccolo, F., & Rebora, A. (2009). Pityriasis rosea: An update with a critical appraisal of its possible herpesviral etiology. *J Am Acad Dermatol*, **61**(2), 303–318.

Friedman, S. J. (1987). Pityriasis rosea with erythema multiforme-like lesions. *J Am Acad Dermatol*, **17**(1), 135–136.

3.1.8 AIDS-Kaposi Sarcoma (HHV-8)

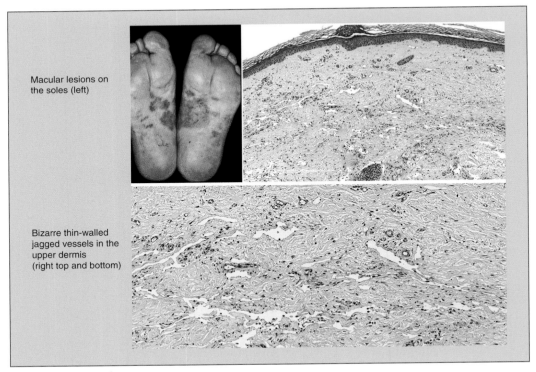

Macular lesions on the soles (left)

Bizarre thin-walled jagged vessels in the upper dermis (right top and bottom)

Figure 3.1.8.1 Kaposi Sarcoma; Patch (Macular) Stage (HHV-8).
Source: Burg et al. (2019). *Atlas of Dermatopathology: Tumors, Nevi, and Cysts* (pp. 298–299). Oxford: Wiley.

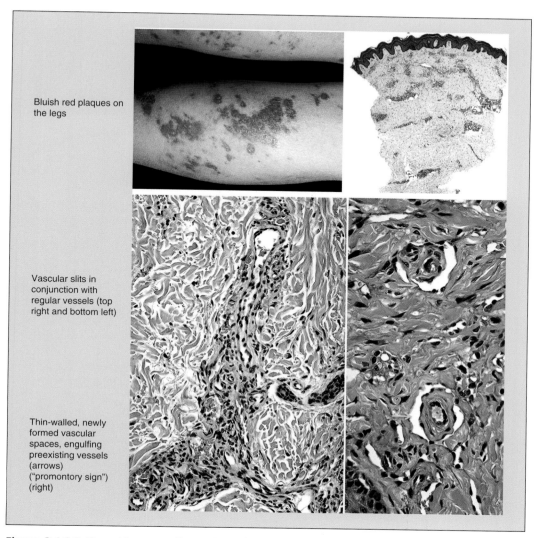

Bluish red plaques on the legs

Vascular slits in conjunction with regular vessels (top right and bottom left)

Thin-walled, newly formed vascular spaces, engulfing preexisting vessels (arrows) ("promontory sign") (right)

Figure 3.1.8.2 Kaposi Sarcoma; Plaque Stage (HHV-8).
Source: Burg et al. (2019). *Atlas of Dermatopathology: Tumors, Nevi, and Cysts* (pp. 298–299). Oxford: Wiley.

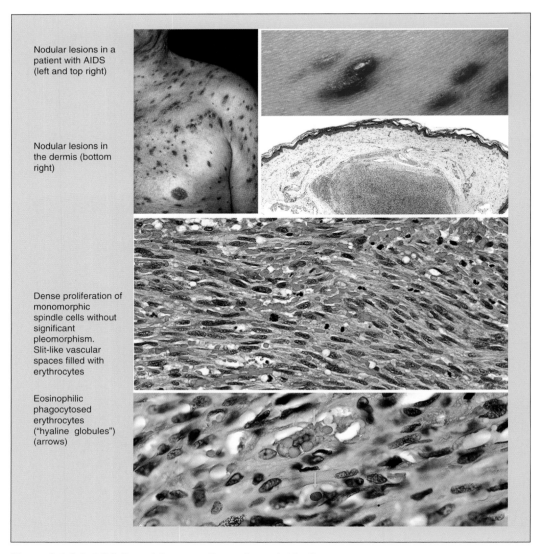

Nodular lesions in a patient with AIDS (left and top right)

Nodular lesions in the dermis (bottom right)

Dense proliferation of monomorphic spindle cells without significant pleomorphism. Slit-like vascular spaces filled with erythrocytes

Eosinophilic phagocytosed erythrocytes ("hyaline globules") (arrows)

Figure 3.1.8.3 AIDS-Kaposi Sarcoma; Tumor Stage (HHV-8).
Source: Burg et al. (2019). *Atlas of Dermatopathology: Tumors, Nevi, and Cysts* (pp. 300–304). Oxford: Wiley.

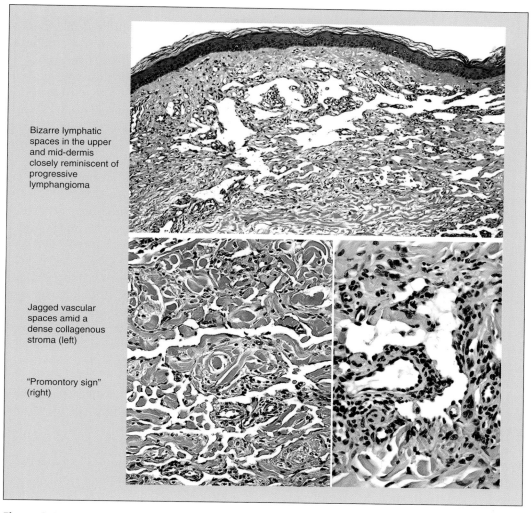

Bizarre lymphatic spaces in the upper and mid-dermis closely reminiscent of progressive lymphangioma

Jagged vascular spaces amid a dense collagenous stroma (left)

"Promontory sign" (right)

Figure 3.1.8.4 Special Feature: AIDS-Kaposi Sarcoma (HHV-8), Lymphangioma-Like Pattern. *Source:* Burg et al. (2019). *Atlas of Dermatopathology: Tumors, Nevi, and Cysts* (pp. 300–304). Oxford: Wiley.

Kaposi sarcoma (KS) is a multicentric vascular tumor of low-grade malignancy, also called a "vascular lesion of indeterminate malignant potential" by some authors, albeit with the potential of classic sarcomatous transformation. Its true origin (blood or lymphatic vessels or pluripotential stem cells) is still under debate, as is its underlying reactive or neoplastic nature. In *WHO Classification of Skin Tumors* (2018), KS has been defined as an "HHV-8 associated vascular proliferation," occurring preferentially in immunocompromised HIV/AIDS patients; "whether it qualifies as a true sarcoma is still a matter of debate."

CF: Under clinical and etiopathogenetic aspects, KS can be subdivided into the following variants: (i) classical/Mediterranean KS; (ii) African-endemic KS; (iii) immunosuppression-associated KS (mostly associated with iatrogenic immunodeficiency in transplant recipients); (iv) epidemic KS (HIV/AIDS–related).

In classic Mediterranean KS, there is a high prevalence of elderly males, with a 15:1 male/female ratio. Most patients are of Jewish or Mediterranean descent. Incipient KS presents with bluish or brown macules and lymphedema, preferably on the lower extremities. Lesions slowly expand, spreading into adjacent anatomical sites. Within months or years, there is transformation of flat lesions into infiltrated plaques and nodules, which finally ulcerate, bleed, and produce exophytic nodular crusted tumors. Mucosal involvement may occur but is rare. Patients often die from KS after the tumor has spread to visceral organs.

In immunodeficiency-associated KS (HIV/AIDS; immunosuppressive therapy; chronic renal failure), small firm red or bluish papules and elongated nodules appear preferentially on the trunk and along skin tension lines and on the mucosa, here initially presenting as multiple patchy bluish enanthems.

HF: The histologic features of all types of KS are identical, albeit with slight differences in chronologic evolution of lesions. While classical KS slowly evolves from macular to plaque and finally to the tumor stage, HIV/AIDS-related KS rapidly produces nodular and exophytic tumors.

- *Patch (Macular) Stage(3.1.8.1):* The histologic picture may be inconspicuous, often suggesting an inflammatory skin condition ("pseudogranulomatous" pattern of KS)
  - Dense and diffuse mixed round cell infiltrate within the upper dermis ("pseudogranulomatous" pattern)
  - Irregular thin-walled vascular spaces between collagen bundles. Regular endothelia co-expressing D2-40/podoplanin and CD34
  - Interstitial hemosiderin deposits and siderophages
  - Plasma cells as a telltale sign of infectious origin

- *Plaque Stage (3.1.8.2):*
  - Involvement of entire reticular dermis: plasma cells, lymphocytes, siderophages and prominent neo-vascularization:
  - Angulated irregular thin-walled small vascular structures and slit-like thin-walled vascular spaces, often "enveloping" preexisting venules and capillaries and adnexal structures ("promontory sign")
  - Focal proliferation of isomorphic spindle cells (CD31+; CD34+; D2-40/podoplanin+; nuclear HHV-8+) arranged as tiny fascicles and strands
  - Mitotic activity; marked lack of pleomorphism
  - Hemorrhage with intra- and extravascular erythrocytes, siderophages, and stacking of erythrocytes
  - Rarely, eosinophilic intracytoplasmic PAS+ hyaline globules (phagocytized erythrocytes) within fusiform tumor cells
  - Dilated lymphatic lacunar spaces with characteristic "stuffing" of intraluminal erythrocytes

- *Nodular/Tumor Stage (3.1.8.3):*
  - Cellular tumor nodules with densely arranged fusiform cells
  - Mitotic activity; lack of nuclear pleomorphism
  - Hyaline intracytoplasmic globules and extracellular stacking of erythrocytes

- Special feature: AIDS-KS (HHV-8), Lymphangioma-Like Pattern *(3.1.8.4)*
  - Bizarre jagged lymphatic spaces in the upper and mid-dermis, suggesting progressive lymphangioma/benign lymphangioendothelioma
  - Very sparse accompanying inflammatory infiltrate
  - Nuclear positivity of endothelial tumor cells for HHV-8 (immunohistochemistry)

DD: Kaposiform hemangioendothelioma; angiosarcoma; epithelioid hemangioendothelioma; pseudomyogenic hemangioendothelioma; hemosiderotic dermatofibroma; acroangiodermatitis Mali (pseudo-Kaposi); benign lymphangioendothelioma/progressive lymphangioma; bacillary angiomatosis; granuloma pyogenicum; spindle cell hemangioma; lymphatic vascular malformations ("hemato-lymphangioma"); malignant melanoma

Reference

Chor, P. J., & Santa Cruz, D. J. (1992). Kaposi's sarcoma. A clinicopathologic review and differential diagnosis. *J Cutan Pathol*, **19**(1), 6–20.

Cossu, S., Satta, R., Cottoni, F., & Massarelli, G. (1997). Lymphangioma-like variant of Kaposi's sarcoma: Clinicopathologic study of seven cases with review of the literature. *Am J Dermatopathol*, **19**(1), 16–22.

Kao, G. F., Johnson, F. B., & Sulica, V. I. (1990). The nature of hyaline (eosinophilic) globules and vascular slits of Kaposi's sarcoma. *Am J Dermatopathol*, **12**(3), 256–267.

McClain, C. M., Haws, A. L., Galfione, S. K., Rapini, R. P., & Hafeez Diwan, A. (2016). Pyogenic granuloma-like Kaposi's sarcoma. *J Cutan Pathol*, **43**(6), 549–551.

O'Donnell, P. J., Pantanowitz, L., & Grayson, W. (2010). Unique histologic variants of cutaneous Kaposi sarcoma. *Am J Dermatopathol*, **32**(3), 244–250.

Ramirez, J. A., Laskin, W. B., & Guitart, J. (2005). Lymphangioma-like Kaposi sarcoma. *J Cutan Pathol*, **32**(4), 286–292.

Sutton, A. M., Tarbox, M., & Burkemper, N. M. (2014). Cavernous hemangioma-like Kaposi sarcoma: A unique histopathologic variant. *Am J Dermatopathol*, **36**(5), 440–442.

Tappero, J. W., Conant, M. A., Wolfe, S. F., & Berger, T. G. (1993). Kaposi's sarcoma. Epidemiology, pathogenesis, histology, clinical spectrum, staging criteria and therapy. *J Am Acad Dermatol*, **28**(3), 371–395.

Yang, S. H., & LeBoit, P. E. (2014). Angiomatous Kaposi sarcoma: A variant that mimics hemangiomas. *Am J Dermatopathol*, **36**(3), 229–237.

Yu, Y., Demierre, M. F., & Mahalingam, M. (2010). Anaplastic Kaposi's sarcoma: An uncommon histologic phenotype with an aggressive clinical course. *J Cutan Pathol*, **37**(10), 1088–1091.

3.1.9 Multicentric Castleman's Disease (HHV-8)

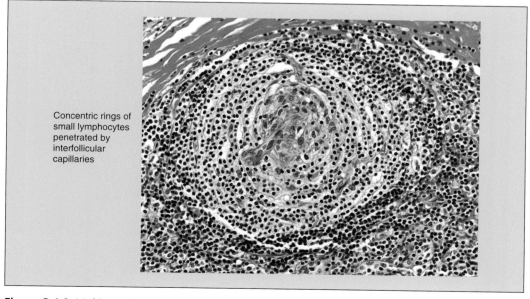

Concentric rings of small lymphocytes penetrated by interfollicular capillaries

Figure 3.1.9 Multicentric Castleman's Disease (HHV-8).

CF: Castleman's disease (CAD) is an unusual lymphoid hyperplasia. The disease may be systemic or localized and can involve lymph nodes and extra nodal sites. Cutaneous CAD characteristically presents with solitary or multiple asymptomatic nodules on the trunk. The plasma cell-rich variant of multicentric CAD in HIV patients is associated with HHV-8.

HF:

- Nodular, well-circumscribed round cell infiltrate in the dermis and subcutis
- Prominent follicular growth pattern with atrophic germinal centers
- Concentric rings of small lymphocytes, penetrated by interfollicular capillaries
- Germinal centers with multinucleated giant cells of the Warthin–Finkeldey type (that are usually encountered in measles)
- Mixed infiltrate of epithelioid histiocytes and lymphoplasmacytoid B-cells. Pronounced vascularity with large numbers of small vessels and thickened hyalinized vessel walls
- The plasma cellular type of CAD contains abundant sheets of mature plasma cells within the interfollicular areas. Subtle hyalinization of vessel walls

DD: Glomeruloid hemangioma; follicular lymphoma.

Reference

Chan, J. K., Fletcher, C. D., Hicklin, G. A., & Rosai, J. (1990). Glomeruloid hemangioma. A distinctive cutaneous lesion of multicentric Castleman's disease associated with POEMS syndrome. *Am J Surg Pathol*, **14**(11), 1036–1046.

Chen, H., Xue, Y., Jiang, Y., Zeng, X., & Sun, J. F. (2012). Cutaneous and systemic plasmacytosis showing histopathologic features as mixed-type Castleman disease: A case report. *Am J Dermatopathol*, **34**(5), 553–556.

Naghashpour, M., Cualing, H. D., Szabunio, M., & Bui, M. M. (2010). Hyaline-vascular Castleman disease: A rare cause of solitary subcutaneous soft tissue mass. *Am J Dermatopathol*, **32**(3), 293–297.

Yang, S. G., Cho, K. H., Bang, Y. J., & Kim, C. W. (1998). A case of glomeruloid hemangioma associated with multicentric Castleman's disease. *Am J Dermatopathol*, **20**(3), 266–270.

3.2 Human Papilloma Virus (HPV)

Various types of HPV are associated with warts.

Type of Wart	HPV Type
Verrucae plantares	1,2,4
Verrucae vulgares	1,2,3,4
Verrucae planae juveniles	3,10
Epidermodysplasia verruciformis	5,8,9,12,14,15,17,19,20,21,47
Condylomata acuminata	6,11
Larynx Papilloma	6,11
Condylomata plana	6,11 und 16,18,31
Bowenoide Papulosis	16, 18 (and seldom 31, 33, 35, 39, 53)
Morbus Heck	13,32

Figure 3.2 Human Papilloma Virus (HPV) Infections.

3.2.1 Verruca Vulgaris

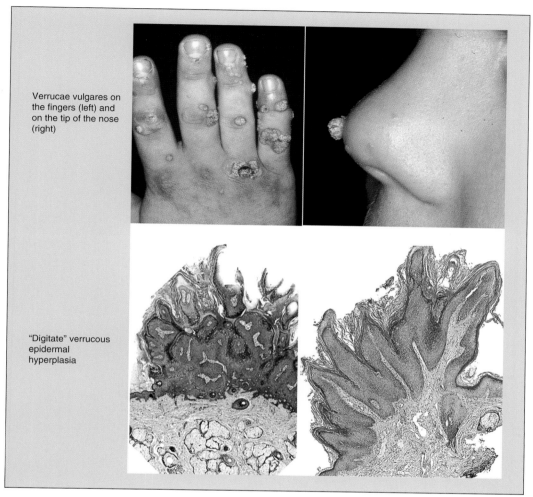

Verrucae vulgares on the fingers (left) and on the tip of the nose (right)

"Digitate" verrucous epidermal hyperplasia

Figure 3.2.1.1 Verruca Vulgaris.
Source: Burg et al. (2015). *Atlas of Dermatopathology: Practical Differential Diagnosis by Clinicopathologic Pattern* (p. 93). Oxford: Wiley.

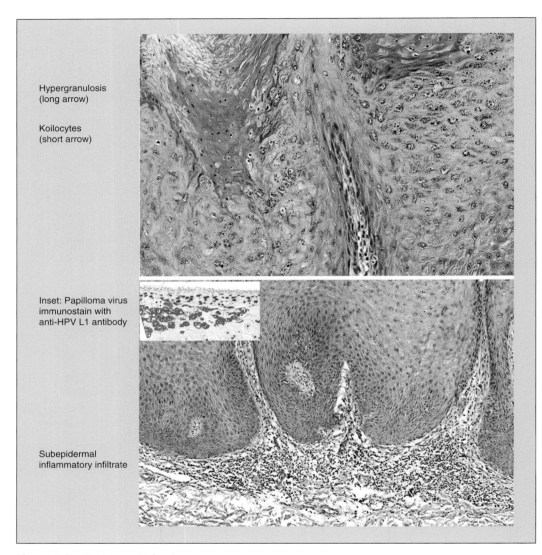

Hypergranulosis
(long arrow)

Koilocytes
(short arrow)

Inset: Papilloma virus
immunostain with
anti-HPV L1 antibody

Subepidermal
inflammatory infiltrate

Figure 3.2.1.2 Verruca Vulgaris.
Source: Burg et al. (2015). *Atlas of Dermatopathology: Practical Differential Diagnosis by Clinicopathologic Pattern* (p. 94). Oxford: Wiley.

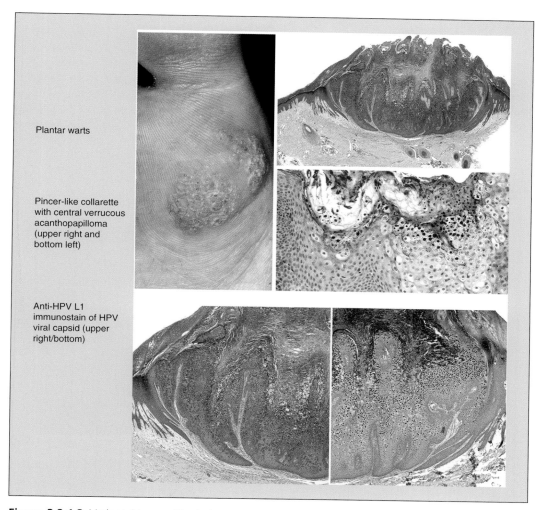

Plantar warts

Pincer-like collarette
with central verrucous
acanthopapilloma
(upper right and
bottom left)

Anti-HPV L1
immunostain of HPV
viral capsid (upper
right/bottom)

Figure 3.2.1.3 Variant: Verruca Plantaris.

Cl: Solitary or grouped papules showing massive hyperkeratosis and sometimes significant inflammation. Depending on the anatomical site, warts may show either endophytic or verrucous-exophytic morphology (verrucae on the soles versus verrucae on the dorsum of the hands).

HF:

- Epidermal hyperplasia with a digitate ("multiple raised fingers") silhouette
- Plantar warts with central papillomatosis and pincer-like acanthosis at the borders
- Hyperkeratosis with focal parakeratosis
- Intracorneal inclusions of hemorrhagic exudate ("papillary body thrombi")
- Hypergranulosis with coarse keratohyalin granules
- Koilocytes ("Bird's-eye" cells) in the granular layer and in the upper stratum spinosum
- Dilated vessels in the papillary dermis
- Inflammatory infiltrate in the upper dermis

DD: Condylomata lata; dyskeratosis follicularis (Darier); syringocystadenoma papilliferum; chronic graft-versus-host disease; acrokeratosis verruciformis.

Reference

Cesinaro, A. M., & Maiorana, A. (2002). Verruca vulgaris with CD30-positive lymphoid infiltrate: A case report. *Am J Dermatopathol*, **24**(3), 260–263.

Fried, I., Kasper, R. S., Hegyi, I., & Kempf, W. (2018). Black dots in palmoplantar warts-challenging a concept: A histopathologic study. *J Am Acad Dermatol*, **79**(2), 380–382.

Park, J. H., Lester, L., Kim, J., & Kwong, B. Y. (2016). Acral verruca-like presentation of chronic graft-vs.-host disease. *J Cutan Pathol*, **43**(3), 236–241.

Xu, X. L., Zhang, G. Y., Zeng, X. S., Wang, Q., & Sun, J. F. (2010). A case of zonal syringocystadenoma papilliferum of the axilla mimicking verruca vulgaris. *Am J Dermatopathol*, **32**(1), 49–51.

3.2.2 Variant: Verrucae Planae

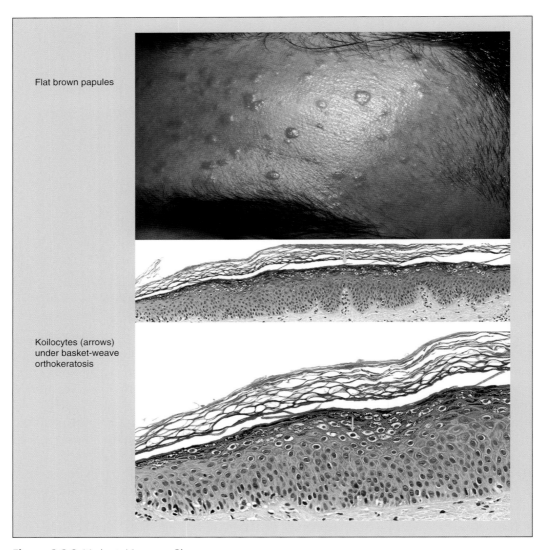

Flat brown papules

Koilocytes (arrows) under basket-weave orthokeratosis

Figure 3.2.2 Variant: Verrucae Planae.
Source: Burg et al. (2015). *Atlas of Dermatopathology: Practical Differential Diagnosis by Clinicopathologic Pattern* (p. 95). Oxford: Wiley.

Cl: Flat, slightly hyperkeratotic papules.
HF:

- Hyperkeratosis
- Moderate acanthosis, but no distinct papillomatosis

- Basket-weave orthokeratosis
- Confluent band of koilocytes ("Bird's-eye" cells) within the granular layer

3.2.3 Variant: Condylomata Acuminata

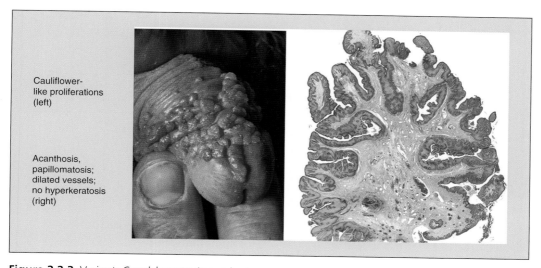

Cauliflower-like proliferations (left)

Acanthosis, papillomatosis; dilated vessels; no hyperkeratosis (right)

Figure 3.2.3 Variant: Condylomata Accuminata.
Source: Burg et al. (2019). *Atlas of Dermatopathology: Tumors, Nevi, and Cysts* (p. 34, 37). Oxford: Wiley.

Cl: Papular and verruciform lesions at anogenital sites.
HF: Acanthopapilloma with focal hyper-parakeratosis and lack of pseudocysts ("naked seborrheic keratosis"). Koilocytes may be present but are extremely sparse.

3.2.4 Differential Diagnosis: Acrokeratosis Verruciformis (Hopf)

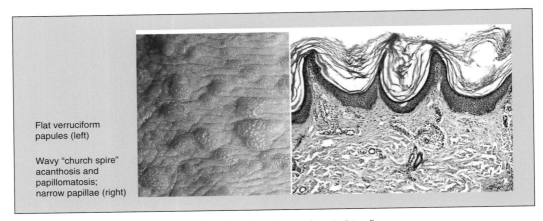

Flat verruciform
papules (left)

Wavy "church spire"
acanthosis and
papillomatosis;
narrow papillae (right)

Figure 3.2.4 Differential Diagnosis: Acrokeratosis Verruciformis (Hopf).

Acrokeratosis verruciformis Hopf is an autosomal dominant genodermatosis closely linked with Darier disease (and also caused by mutations in the *SERCA2-ATPase* gene) in which multiple papules, resembling plane warts, develop on the dorsa of the hands and fingers and to a lesser extent on the feet, forearms, and legs. Lesions identical to those of idiopathic acrokeratosis verruciformis occur in patients with Darier's disease (AVH and DD as allelic disorders) or with epidermodysplasia verruciformis. In the latter, relationship with HPV infection has been discussed.

Cl: Multiple flat hyperkeratotic papules on peripheral parts of the limbs (dorsa of the hands, feet, forearms).

HF:

- Orthohyperkeratosis
- Wavy (church spire) acanthosis
- Papillomatosis
- Thinned papillae

Reference

Bergman, R., Sezin, T., Indelman, M., Helou, W. A., & Avitan-Hersh, E. (2012). Acrokeratosis verruciformis of Hopf showing P602L mutation in ATP2A2 and overlapping histopathological features with Darier disease. *Am J Dermatopathol*, **34**(6), 597–601.

Matsumoto, A., Gregory, N., Rady, P. L., Tyring, S. K., & Carlson, J. A. (2017). Brief report: HPV-17 infection in Darier disease with acrokeratosis verrucosis of Hopf. *Am J Dermatopathol*, **39**(5), 370–373.

3.2.5 Bowenoid Papulosis

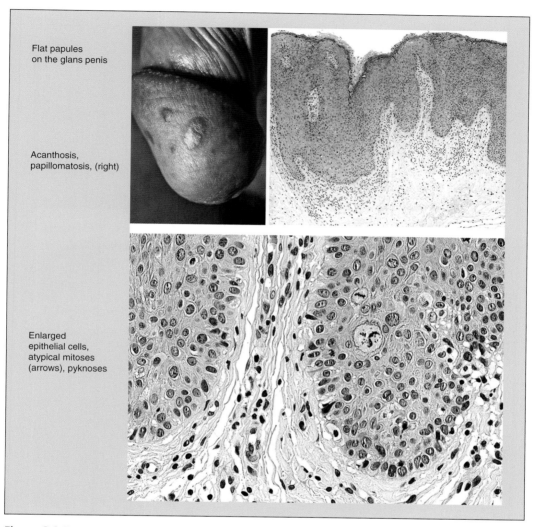

Flat papules
on the glans penis

Acanthosis,
papillomatosis, (right)

Enlarged
epithelial cells,
atypical mitoses
(arrows), pyknoses

Figure 3.2.5 Bowenoid Papulosis.
Source: Burg et al. (2019). *Atlas of Dermatopathology: Tumors, Nevi, and Cysts* (p. 35, 36). Oxford: Wiley.

Cl: Solitary or confluent flat papular eruptions in anogenital localization, often associated with high-risk oncogenic HPV infection (HPV16, HPV18).
HF: Scattered atypical epithelial cells with nuclear pleomorphism and mitotic activity. Positivity for p16. Often with increased melanin.

Reference

Kazlouskaya, V., Shustef, E., Allam, S. H., Lal, K., & Elston, D. (2013). Expression of p16 protein in lesional and perilesional condyloma acuminata and bowenoid papulosis: Clinical significance and diagnostic implications. *J Am Acad Dermatol*, **69**(3), 444–449.

3.2.6 Epidermodysplasia Verruciformis (Lewandowsky–Lutz); Verrucosis Generalisata

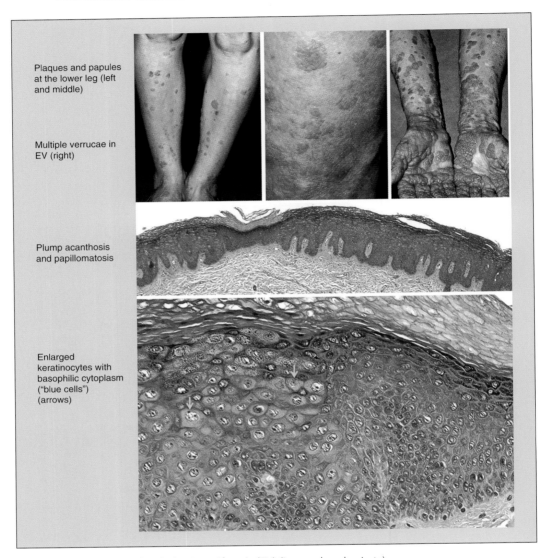

Plaques and papules at the lower leg (left and middle)

Multiple verrucae in EV (right)

Plump acanthosis and papillomatosis

Enlarged keratinocytes with basophilic cytoplasm ("blue cells") (arrows)

Figure 3.2.6 Epidermodysplasia Verruciformis (EV) (Lewandowsky–Lutz).

In a minority of patients with EV, there is autosomal recessive inheritance, while most cases of EV are sporadic. EV is associated with oncogenic HPV infection (EV-types of HPV) and may progress to squamous cell carcinoma.

Cl: Circumscribed small confluent plaques, mostly on sun-exposed sites. Lesions may either be flat and resemble pityriasis versicolor, or more lichenoid, resembling plane warts. The mucosa is spared.

HF: Intraepidermal enlarged keratinocytes with swollen and smudged bluish cytoplasm (basophilic "blue cells" as a telltale sign). Dyskeratotic and pyknotic cells may be present in small numbers. Detection of beta-HPV types by PCR.

DD: Squamous cell carcinoma; seborrheic keratosis.

Reference

Champagne, C., Moore, L., Reule, R., Dyer, J. A., Rady, P., Tyring, S. K., & North, J. P. (2015). Cornoid lamella-like structures in HIV-associated Epidermodysplasia verruciformis: A unique histopathologic finding. *Am J Dermatopathol*, **37**(12), 929–932.

Collins, M. K., Peters, K., English, J. C., 3rd, Rady, P., Tyring, S., & Jedrych, J. (2018). Cutaneous squamous cell carcinoma with epidermodysplasia verruciformis-like features in a patient with Schimke immune-osseous dysplasia. *J Cutan Pathol*, **45**(6), 465–467.

Morrison, C., Eliezri, Y., Magro, C., & Nuovo, G. J. (2002). The histologic spectrum of epidermodysplasia verruciformis in transplant and AIDS patients. *J Cutan Pathol*, **29**(8), 480–489.

Tomasini, C., Aloi, F., & Pippione, M. (1993). Seborrheic keratosis-like lesions in epidermodysplasia verruciformis. *J Cutan Pathol*, **20**(3), 237–241.

3.3 Viral Exanthema

Viral exanthema present with a plethora of cutaneous lesions, some of them suggesting allergic or reactive conditions. Traditional taxonomy of viral eruptions originally comprised six viral exanthems ("the six diseases"): Measles, scarlet fever, German measles, rubeola scarlatinosa, erythema infectiosum, and exanthema subitum. This classification is obsolete – but the underlying problem remains: The diagnoses of these six viral exanthema are usually made clinically rather than histologically and are difficult to differentiate from each other by the inexperienced eye.

3.3.1 Measles

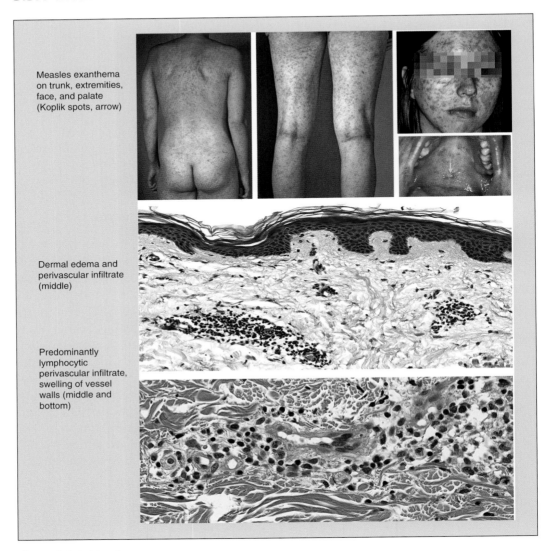

Measles exanthema on trunk, extremities, face, and palate (Koplik spots, arrow)

Dermal edema and perivascular infiltrate (middle)

Predominantly lymphocytic perivascular infiltrate, swelling of vessel walls (middle and bottom)

Figure 3.3.1 Measles.

Measles is caused by an RNA paramyxovirus. Non-vaccinated young children are at a particularly high risk of infection due to the high contagious potential of the measles virus.

CF: Following a prodromal phase with fever and general malaise, skin lesions appear as a generalized eruption of red macules and papules, starting behind the ears and spreading to the face, neck, trunk, and extremities. Lesions may get hemorrhagic. Mucosal involvement is common: typical Koplik spots on the palate are a telltale sign of measles infection.

HF:

• Follicular necrotic keratinocytes and small intraepidermal clusters of folliculocentric necrotic keratinocytes are the leading histopathological criterion of measles virus infection

- The cytoplasm of these necrotic keratinocytes stains positive with anti-measles antibody (immunohistochemistry)
- Dermal edema, rarely associated with lymphocytic vasculitis and hemorrhage; with diffuse scarce infiltrate composed of lymphocytes, eosinophils, plasma cells. Multinucleated giant cells (Warthin–Finkeldey cells) in the lymph node; similar cells may be present in the epidermis

DD: Drug eruptions; other viral exanthema.

Reference

Sidhu, H. K., Lanoue, J., Nazarian, R., Mercer, S. E., Gordon, R. E., & Phelps, R. G. (2015). Histopathology of measles: Report of 2 cases with new findings. *Am J Dermatopathol,* **37**(7), 563–566.

Liersch, J., Omaj, R., & Schaller, J. (2019). Histopathological and immunohistochemical characteristics of measles exanthema: A study of a series of 13 adult cases and review of the literature. *Am J Dermatopathol,* **41**(12), 914–992.

Magdaleno-Tapial, J., Valenzuela-Onate, C., Giacaman-von der Weth, M., Ferrer-Guillen, B., Garcia-Legaz Martinez, M., Martinez-Domenech, A., … Alegre-de Miquel, V. (2019). Follicle and sebaceous gland multinucleated cells in measles. *Am J Dermatopathol,* **41**(4), 289–292.

Tirado, M., Adamzik, K., & Boer-Auer, A. (2015). Follicular necrotic keratinocytes – a helpful clue to the diagnosis of measles. *J Cutan Pathol,* **42**(9), 632–638.

3.4 Parvovirus Infections and Coxsackievirus Infections

3.4.1 Erythema Infectiosum; (Slapped Cheek Disease; Fifth Disease)

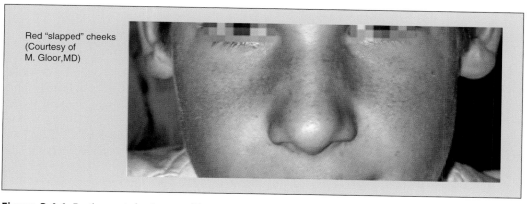

Red "slapped" cheeks
(Courtesy of
M. Gloor,MD)

Figure 3.4.1 Erythema Infectiosum; (Slapped Cheek Disease; Fifth Disease).

CF: Parvovirus B19 (PVB19) infection causes confluent livedo reticularis-like gyrate erythema on the cheeks, followed by gyrate and wreath-like erythema on the arms.

HF°: Sparse perivascular lymphocytic infiltrate in the upper dermal plexus. No vasculitis.

DD: Drug eruptions; other viral exanthemas.

3.4.2 Papular Purpuric Gloves-and-Socks Syndrome

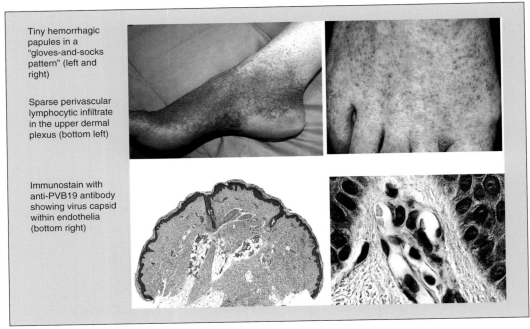

Tiny hemorrhagic papules in a "gloves-and-socks pattern" (left and right)

Sparse perivascular lymphocytic infiltrate in the upper dermal plexus (bottom left)

Immunostain with anti-PVB19 antibody showing virus capsid within endothelia (bottom right)

Figure 3.4.2 Gloves-and-Socks Sndrome. *Source:* Courtesy of L. Requena,MD, Madrid.

CF: Parvovirus B19-induced eruption of confluent small erythematous and purpuric papules at body sites that are often covered by gloves and socks, preferentially palms and soles and adjacent marginal skin ("gloves-and-socks" pattern of cutaneous lesions).

HF: Sparse perivascular lymphocytic infiltrate in the upper dermal plexus, often associated with slight lymphocytic vasculitis and discrete extravasation of erythrocytes. Remarkably, immunohistochemistry may show intracytoplasmic viral deposits within endothelia and – rarely – adjacent round cells. PCR from lesional skin may be misleading (high percentage of false positives) as majority of patients has had prior PVB19 infection and is harboring virus in the blood.

DD: Drug eruptions; other viral exanthema.

Reference

Cioc, A. M., Sedmak, D. D., Nuovo, G. J., Dawood, M. R., Smart, G., & Magro, C. M. (2002). Parvovirus B19 associated adult Henoch Schonlein purpura. *J Cutan Pathol,* **29**(10), 602–607.

Harms, M., Feldmann, R., & Saurat, J. H. (1990). Papular-purpuric "gloves and socks" syndrome. *J Am Acad Dermatol,* **23**(5 Pt 1), 850–854.

Santonja, C., Nieto-Gonzalez, G., Santos-Briz, A., Gutierrez Zufiaurre Mde, L., Cerroni, L., Kutzner, H., & Requena, L. (2011). Immunohistochemical detection of parvovirus B19 in "gloves and socks" papular purpuric syndrome: Direct evidence for viral endothelial involvement. Report of three cases and review of the literature. *Am J Dermatopathol,* **33**(8), 790–795.

Smith, S. B., Libow, L. F., Elston, D. M., Bernert, R. A., & Warschaw, K. E. (2002). Gloves and socks syndrome: Early and late histopathologic features. *J Am Acad Dermatol,* **47**(5), 749–754.

3.4.3 Hand-Foot-and-Mouth Disease (Coxsackie Virus)

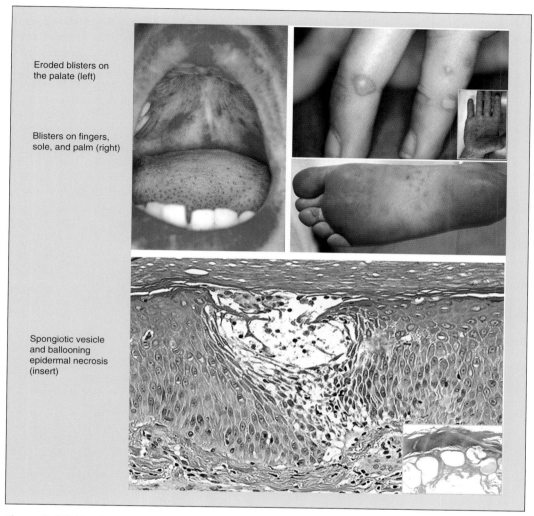

Eroded blisters on the palate (left)

Blisters on fingers, sole, and palm (right)

Spongiotic vesicle and ballooning epidermal necrosis (insert)

Figure 3.4.3 Hand-Foot-and-Mouth Disease.
Source: Burg et al. (2015). *Atlas of Dermatopathology: Practical Differential Diagnosis by Clinicopathologic Pattern* (p. 91). Oxford: Wiley.

The highly contagious disease caused by *Coxsackievirus A16* commonly affects children and adolescents. The highly contagious *Coxsackie virus A16* is a member of the Picornaviridae family of small RNA viruses. *Enterovirus 71* and others may induce identical clinical symptoms.

CF: The infection primarily involves palms, soles, buttocks, and palate with conspicuous intact blisters at the acral sites and eroded erythematous lesions on the mucous membrane. The buttocks may show eruptive small vesicles with rapid subsequent erosion. There may be a slight accompanying fever, but patients generally do not feel sick.

HF:

- Spongiosis with conspicuous reticular epithelial degeneration showing elongated ("stretched") keratinocytes amidst massive intercellular edema
- "Stretching" and ballooning (intracytoplasmic edema) of epidermal cells
- Spongiotic blister formation
- Absence of distinct necroses and pyknoses
- Edema in the papillary dermis with lymphocytic infiltrate; without vasculopathic changes

DD: Herpes simplex; varicella; erythema multiforme; dyshidrosiform (allergic) eruption.

3.5 Polyoma Virus Infections

3.5.1 Trichodysplasia Spinulosa

Reference

Boer-Auer, A., & Metze, D. (2019). Histopathology of hand-foot-mouth disease in adults and criteria for differentiation from erythema multiforme. *Am J Dermatopathol,* **41**(4), 273–280.

Herrero, M., Kutzner, H., Fraga, J., & Llamas-Velasco, M. (2019). Immunohistochemical study of 2 cases of Coxsackie A6-induced atypical hand-foot-and-mouth disease. *Am J Dermatopathol,* **41**(10), 741–743.

Second, J., Velter, C., Cales, S., Truchetet, F., Lipsker, D., & Cribier, B. (2017). Clinicopathologic analysis of atypical hand, foot, and mouth disease in adult patients. *J Am Acad Dermatol,* **76**(4), 722–729.

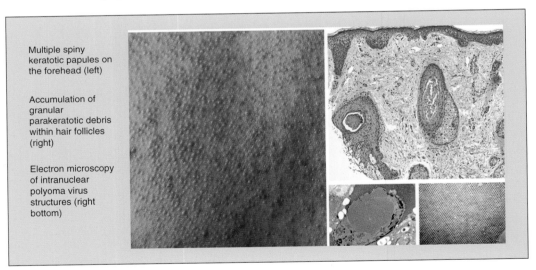

Multiple spiny keratotic papules on the forehead (left)

Accumulation of granular parakeratotic debris within hair follicles (right)

Electron microscopy of intranuclear polyoma virus structures (right bottom)

Figure 3.5.1.1 Trichodysplasia Spinulosa.

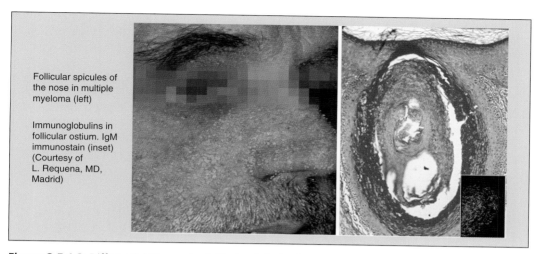

Follicular spicules of the nose in multiple myeloma (left)

Immunoglobulins in follicular ostium. IgM immunostain (inset) (Courtesy of L. Requena, MD, Madrid)

Figure 3.5.1.2 Differential Diagnosis: Follicular Spicules in Myeloma (Nazzaro Syndrome).

This rare folliculocentric cutaneous disease is commonly associated with human polyoma virus infection (Trichodysplasia spinulosa human polyoma virus/Ts-HPyV) in immunocompromised patients.

CF: Small, follicle-bound, spiny, keratotic papules mostly on the face, resembling fine hairs or follicular spicules. Subsequently, eyebrows and eyelashes disappear due to destruction of hair follicle epithelium.

HF:

- Granular hair shafts with coarse keratohyalin granules
- Accumulation of granular parakeratotic debris within hair follicle
- Disorganized eosinophilic inner root sheath cells with few necrotic keratinocytes
- Conspicuously large trichohyalin granules within keratinocytes of inner root sheath

DD: Warts; keratosis pilaris; ulerythema ophryogenes; follicular spicules of the nose, associated with multiple myeloma (paraneoplastic (Nazzaro) syndrome).

Reference

Elaba, Z., Hughey, L., Isayeva, T., Weeks, B., Solovan, C., Solovastru, L., & Andea, A. (2012). Ultrastructural and molecular confirmation of the trichodysplasia spinulosa-associated polyomavirus in biopsies of patients with trichodysplasia spinulosa. *J Cutan Pathol,* **39**(11), 1004–1009.

Kadam, P., Pan, T., Gates, R., Rivetz, J., Rady, P., Tyring, S., & Carlson, J. A. (2017). Detection of beta-human papillomavirus in a child with polyomavirus-associated trichodysplasia spinulosa. *Am J Dermatopathol,* **39**(12), 928–931.

Kaddu, S., Soyer, H. P., & Kerl, H. (1995). Palmar filiform hyperkeratosis: A new paraneoplastic syndrome? *J Am Acad Dermatol,* **33**(2 Pt 2), 337–340.

Matthews, M. R., Wang, R. C., Reddick, R. L., Saldivar, V. A., & Browning, J. C. (2011). Viral-associated trichodysplasia spinulosa: A case with electron microscopic and molecular detection of the trichodysplasia spinulosa-associated human polyomavirus. *J Cutan Pathol,* **38**(5), 420–431.

Nazzaro, P., Argentieri, R., Balus, L., Bassetti, F., Fazio, M., Giacalone, B., & Ponno, R. (1974). [Paraneoplastic syndrome with papulo-keratosic lesions of the extremities and diffuse spinulose pilar keratosis]. *Ann Dermatol Syphiligr (Paris),* **101**(4), 411–413.

Paul, C., Fermand, J. P., Flageul, B., Caux, F., Duterque, M., Dubertret, L., & Aractingi, S. (1995). Hyperkeratotic spicules and monoclonal gammopathy. *J Am Acad Dermatol,* **33**(2 Pt 2), 346–351.

Requena, L., Sarasa, J. L., Ortiz Masllorens, F., Martin, L., Pique, E., Olivares, M., ... Gomez Octavio, J. (1995). Follicular spicules of the nose: A peculiar cutaneous manifestation of multiple myeloma with cryoglobulinemia. *J Am Acad Dermatol, 32*(5 Pt 2), 834–839.

3.5.2 Merkel Cell Carcinoma (Primary Neuroendocrine Carcinoma of the Skin; Trabecular Carcinoma of Toker)

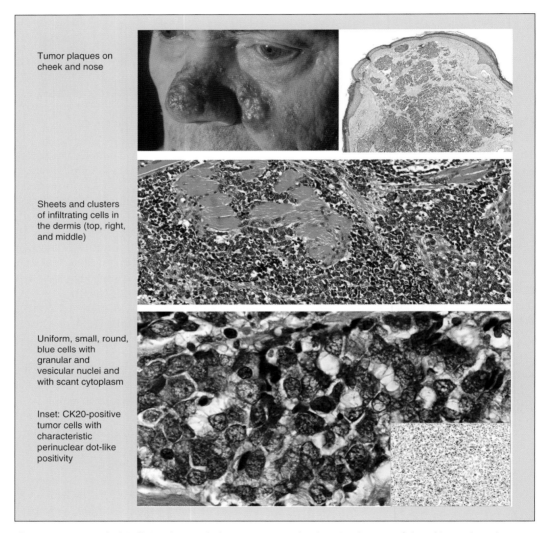

Tumor plaques on cheek and nose

Sheets and clusters of infiltrating cells in the dermis (top, right, and middle)

Uniform, small, round, blue cells with granular and vesicular nuclei and with scant cytoplasm

Inset: CK20-positive tumor cells with characteristic perinuclear dot-like positivity

Figure 3.5.2 Merkel Cell Carcinoma (Primary Neuroendocrine Carcinoma of the Skin; Trabecular Carcinoma of Toker).
Source: Burg et al. (2019). *Atlas of Dermatopathology: Tumors, Nevi, and Cysts* (pp. 360, 361). Oxford: Wiley.

The so-called Merkel cells of Merkel cell carcinoma (MCC) are neoplastic epithelial cells of neuroendocrine origin – most likely unrelated to autochthonous intraepidermal Merkel cells. Although it has been suggested that MCC might originate from autochthonous follicle-bound genuine Merkel cells, this hypothesis has not yet been unequivocally proved. About half of all cutaneous MCCs harbor Merkel cell polyomavirus (MCPyV), which belongs to the family of human polyoma viruses (HPyV). The other half of cutaneous MCCs is MCPyV-negative and often shows morphological overlap with conventional squamous cell carcinoma (hybrid variants of MCC).

Cl: The sun-exposed head and neck sites of elderly patients are most commonly affected by this highly aggressive, dome-shaped, rapidly growing, and infiltrating tumor, which shows early metastases to regional lymph nodes and visceral organs.

HF:

• Dermal nodular sheets and clusters of darkly basophilic round tumor cells without distinct borders. Arrangement mostly in sheets, occasionally in a trabecular pattern. Often suggesting high-grade cutaneous B-cell lymphoma

• Predominance of monomorphous large hyperchromatic round basophilic tumor cells with smudged cytoplasmic borders

• Tumor sheets interspersed with numerous mitoses and apoptoses

• Focal squamous transformation (SCC) in about half of the cases

• Azzopardi phenomenon (i.e. basophilic granular nuclear DNA lacing the walls of small vessels), which is typically found in small cell carcinoma of the lungs, is lacking in cutaneous MCC

• Immunophenotype: expression of neurofilament, CK20 (dot-like intracytoplasmic pattern), CAM5.2, chromogranin, synaptophysin, InsM1 (found in all carcinomas of neuroendocrine origin); BerEP4 (also expressed in BCCs)

DD: High-grade cutaneous (B-cell) lymphoma; B-CLL; other primary and secondary cutaneous neuroendocrine carcinomas; metastasizing lung carcinoma; sweat gland carcinoma; squamous cell carcinoma; basal cell carcinoma; Bowen's disease; melanoma.

Reference

Bandino, J. P., Purvis, C. G., Shaffer, B. R., Gad, A., & Elston, D. M. (2018). A comparison of the histopathologic growth patterns between non-merkel cell small round blue cell tumors and Merkel cell carcinoma. *Am J Dermatopathol*, **40**(11), 815–818.

Feng, H., Shuda, M., Chang, Y., & Moore, P. S. (2008). Clonal integration of a polyomavirus in human Merkel cell carcinoma. *Science*, **319**(5866), 1096–1100.

Heath, M., Jaimes, N., Lemos, B., Mostaghimi, A., Wang, L. C., Penas, P. F., & Nghiem, P. (2008). Clinical characteristics of Merkel cell carcinoma at diagnosis in 195 patients: The AEIOU features. *J Am Acad Dermatol*, **58**(3), 375–381.

Hwang, J. H., Alanen, K., Dabbs, K. D., Danyluk, J., & Silverman, S. (2008). Merkel cell carcinoma with squamous and sarcomatous differentiation. *J Cutan Pathol*, **35**(10), 955–959.

Jackson, C. R., & Linos, K. (2019). SOX10 dot-like paranuclear positivity in Merkel cell carcinoma: Report of 2 cases. *Am J Dermatopathol*, **41**(9), 694–695.

Koba, S., Nagase, K., Ikeda, S., Aoki, S., Misago, N., & Narisawa, Y. (2015). Merkel cell carcinoma with glandular differentiation admixed with sweat gland carcinoma and spindle cell carcinoma: Histogenesis of Merkel cell carcinoma from hair follicle stem cells. *Am J Dermatopathol*, **37**(3), e31–36.

Le, M. D., O'Steen, L. H., & Cassarino, D. S. (2017). A rare case of CK20/CK7 double negative Merkel cell carcinoma. *Am J Dermatopathol*, **39**(3), 208–211.

Miraflor, A. P., LeBoit, P. E., & Hirschman, S. A. (2016). Intraepidermal Merkel cell carcinoma with pagetoid Bowen's disease. *J Cutan Pathol*, **43**(11), 921–926.

Mitteldorf, C., Mertz, K. D., Fernandez-Figueras, M. T., Schmid, M., Tronnier, M., & Kempf, W. (2012). Detection of Merkel cell polyomavirus and human papillomaviruses in Merkel cell carcinoma combined with squamous cell carcinoma in immunocompetent European patients. *Am J Dermatopathol*, **34**(5), 506–510.

Succaria, F., Radfar, A., & Bhawan, J. (2014). Merkel cell carcinoma (primary neuroendocrine carcinoma of skin) mimicking basal cell carcinoma with review of different histopathologic features. *Am J Dermatopathol*, **36**(2), 160–166.

Veija, T., Kero, M., Koljonen, V., & Bohling, T. (2019). ALK and EGFR expression by immunohistochemistry are associated with Merkel cell polyomavirus status in Merkel cell carcinoma. *Histopathology*, **74**(6), 829–835.

3.6 Poxviruses

Poxviruses are large complex DNA viruses, comprising the family of orthopox viruses (cowpox/catpox, monkey pox, vaccinia, and variola), parapoxviruses (ecthyma contagiosum/orf and milker's nodule), and molluscum pox viruses.

3.6.1 Orthopox Virus Infections

Orthopox virus infections have clinical and histological features in common. Differences may be subtle.

Clinically, there usually is erythematous swelling at the site of inoculation with a papulovesicular eruption, evolving into umbilicated pustules with focal hemorrhagic necrosis and crust formation.

Histologically, in acute lesions, there is prominent reticular degeneration and necrosis of the epidermis, ballooning, and necrosis of keratinocytes. Blister formation may be minimal. Multinucleated giant cells can be present. Accompanying papillary edema with erythrocyte extravasation and inflammatory infiltrate consisting of lymphocytes, neutrophils, and eosinophils is seen in the upper and mid-dermis.

DD: Due to their significant morphological overlap, poxvirus infections are exceedingly difficult to differentiate from each other (e.g. variola vera versus monkey pox). Advanced molecular diagnostic methods (PCR; sequencing methodology; electron microscopy/negative staining) in conjunction with clinical and historical data are mandatory. Remarkably, poxviruses, in particular monkey pox, are endemic in large parts of Africa (Democratic Republic of the Congo); acute infections with monkey pox may mimic variola vera; impetigo contagiosa; dermatitis due to mites; varicella; pustula maligna (anthrax).

Reference

Asiran Serdar, Z., Yasar, S., Demirkesen, C., & Aktas Karabay, E. (2018). Poxvirus-induced vascular angiogenesis mimicking pyogenic granuloma. *Am J Dermatopathol*, **40**(9), e126–129.

Molina-Ruiz, A. M., Santonja, C., Rutten, A., Cerroni, L., Kutzner, H., & Requena, L. (2015). Immunohistochemistry in the diagnosis of cutaneous viral infections- part II: Cutaneous viral infections by parvoviruses, poxviruses, paramyxoviridae, picornaviridae, retroviruses and filoviruses. *Am J Dermatopathol*, **37**(2), 93–106.

3.6.1.1 Cowpox (Catpox)

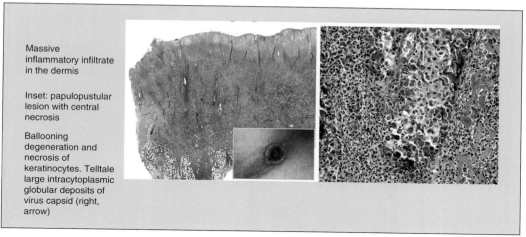

Massive inflammatory infiltrate in the dermis

Inset: papulopustular lesion with central necrosis

Ballooning degeneration and necrosis of keratinocytes. Telltale large intracytoplasmic globular deposits of virus capsid (right, arrow)

Figure 3.6.1.1 Cowpox (Catpox).

Field voles, rats, and mice are the natural reservoir of the virus. Transmission to humans occurs via cats or directly via rats that are kept by young people as pets. Remarkably, a high percentage of cats harbor not only cowpox virus but also Bartonella under their claws and consequently are a great infectious peril for immunocompromised people. Symptoms include a mild fever and lymphadenopathy. Rarely, lesions may present with massive edema, erythema, focal blistering, and large black eschars. Involvement of the conjunctivae is particularly dangerous and often clinically missed. Deer pox (in hunters) may cause identical symptoms.

Reference

Nasemann, T., Mayr, A., Schaeg, G., Kimmig, W., & Mahnel, H. (1987). [Cowpox virus infection in a young girl]. *Hautarzt*, **38**(7), 414–418.

Wienecke, R., Wolff, H., Schaller, M., Meyer, H., & Plewig, G. (2000). Cowpox virus infection in an 11-year-old girl. *J Am Acad Dermatol*, **42**(5 Pt 2), 892–894.

3.6.1.2 Vaccinia Inoculata

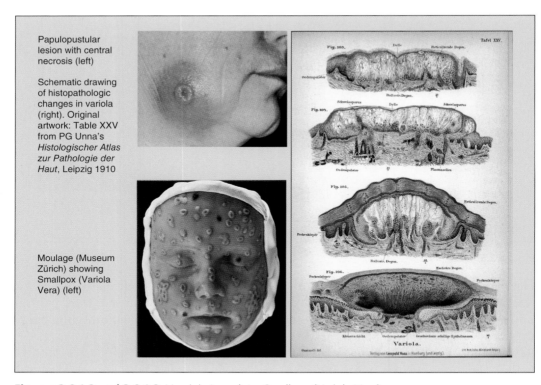

Papulopustular lesion with central necrosis (left)

Schematic drawing of histopathologic changes in variola (right). Original artwork: Table XXV from PG Unna's *Histologischer Atlas zur Pathologie der Haut*, Leipzig 1910

Moulage (Museum Zürich) showing Smallpox (Variola Vera) (left)

Figures 3.6.1.2 and 3.6.1.3 Vaccinia Inoculata; Smallpox (Variola Vera).

History of previous poxvirus vaccination. General dissemination of vaccinia virus preferentially occurs in patients with atopic dermatitis, evolving into eczema vaccinatum.

Reference

Landthaler, M., Strasser, S., & Schmoeckel, C. (1988). [Vaccinia inoculata]. *Hautarzt*, **39**(5), 322–323.

3.6.1.3 Smallpox (Variola Vera)

Smallpox is highly contagious and often a lethal disease caused by *Poxvirus variola*. Smallpox has been eradicated according to the 1980 declaration of the World Health Organization (WHO); albeit, virus strains are kept for research purposes by the Centers of Disease Control and Russian laboratories. Remarkably, clinical and histopathological symptoms of monkey pox (Democratic Republic of the Congo) and variola vera overlap. Consequently, thorough clinical and diagnostic vigilance is paramount.

The clinical course is severe and associated with general malaise from the beginning of the infection. The umbilicated lesions appear and mature simultaneously, sequentially producing papules, vesicles, pustules, crusts, finally leaving typical umbilicated "varioliform" scars with eschars. Marked involvement of face, scalp, palms, and soles with sparing of axillae and groins is typical.

Reference

Nuovo, G. J., Plaza, J. A., & Magro, C. (2003). Rapid diagnosis of smallpox infection and differentiation from its mimics. *Diagn Mol Pathol*, **12**(2), 103–107.

3.6.2 Parapox Virus Infections
3.6.2.1 Ecthyma Contagiosum (Orf)

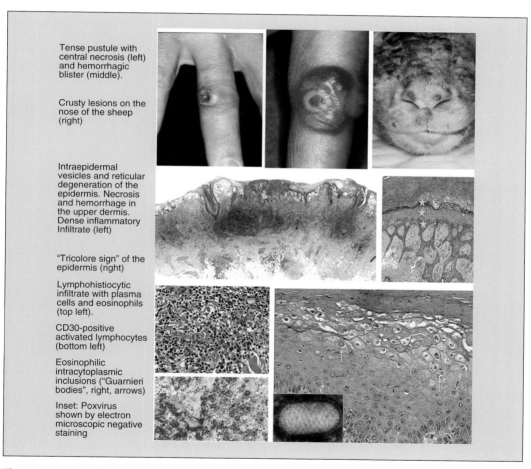

Tense pustule with central necrosis (left) and hemorrhagic blister (middle).

Crusty lesions on the nose of the sheep (right)

Intraepidermal vesicles and reticular degeneration of the epidermis. Necrosis and hemorrhage in the upper dermis. Dense inflammatory Infiltrate (left)

"Tricolore sign" of the epidermis (right)

Lymphohistiocytic infiltrate with plasma cells and eosinophils (top left).

CD30-positive activated lymphocytes (bottom left)

Eosinophilic intracytoplasmic inclusions ("Guarnieri bodies", right, arrows)

Inset: Poxvirus shown by electron microscopic negative staining

Figure 3.6.2.1 Ecthyma Contagiosum (Orf).

The causative agent is *Parapoxvirus ovis (orf virus)*. Goats, sheep, and lambs are the natural reservoir of the virus. Infection occurs via direct animal contact (shepherds, butchers). **CF**: Marked erythematous swelling at the site of inoculation with erythema and iris-like edematous blister formation, often hemorrhagic and crusted, followed by eschar formation.

HF:

- Reticular degeneration of upper parts of epidermis with telltale "tricolore sign" showing blue-white-red tinged epidermal layers
- Marked ballooning of keratinocytes
- Eosinophilic intracytoplasmic inclusions of virus capsid in keratinocytes (Guarnieri bodies)
- Necrosis and hemorrhage (late)

- Dermal round cell infiltrate, often studded with multiple CD30-positive lymphocytes and CD123-positive plasmacytoid dendritic cells (remarkably an almost identical immunophenotype may be found in inflamed molluscum contagiosum)
- Excessive neovascularization of densely packed capillaries and venules may occur beneath the lesion, often suggesting a benign vascular tumor

DD: Erythema multiforme; milker's nodule; pyogenic granuloma.

Reference

Asiran Serdar, Z., Yasar, S., Demirkesen, C., & Aktas Karabay, E. (2018). Poxvirus-induced vascular angiogenesis mimicking pyogenic granuloma. *Am J Dermatopathol*, **40**(9), e126–129.

3.6.2.2 Variant: Milker's Nodule

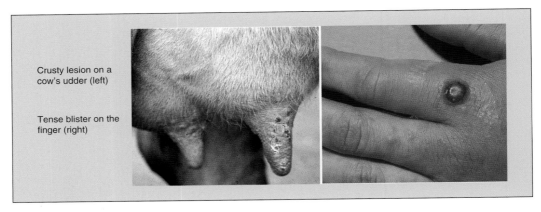

Crusty lesion on a cow's udder (left)

Tense blister on the finger (right)

Figure 3.6.2.2 Variant: Milker's Nodule.

Milker's nodule may be considered as a morphological variant of orf. This parapox virus is transferred via direct contact from cow's udder to the farmer's finger. The virus is not identical with "cowpox" virus (the latter is a misnomer: cowpox virus should be termed field-vole virus).

CF: Small brown nodule or multiple nodules with whitish central necrosis at the site of inoculation. Moderate inflammation.

HF: Ecthyma contagiosum (orf)

- Reticular epidermal degeneration and vesicle formation in the acanthotic epidermis
- Ballooning of keratinocytes with Guarnieri bodies
- Giant cells and inclusions in keratinocytes may occasionally be absent
- Edema and mixed cellular inflammatory infiltrate in the dermis, occasionally simulating CD30-positive lymphoproliferation
- Prominent postcapillary venules

DD: Ecthyma contagiosum; insect bite; bacterial folliculitis.

Reference

Werchniak, A. E., Herfort, O. P., Farrell, T. J., Connolly, K. S., & Baughman, R. D. (2003).

Milker's nodule in a healthy young woman. *J Am Acad Dermatol*, **49**(5), 910–911.

Werner, B., Massone, C., Kerl, H., & Cerroni, L. (2008). Large CD30-positive cells in benign, atypical lymphoid infiltrates of the skin. *J Cutan Pathol*, **35**(12), 1100–1107.

3.6.2.3 Molluscum Contagiosum

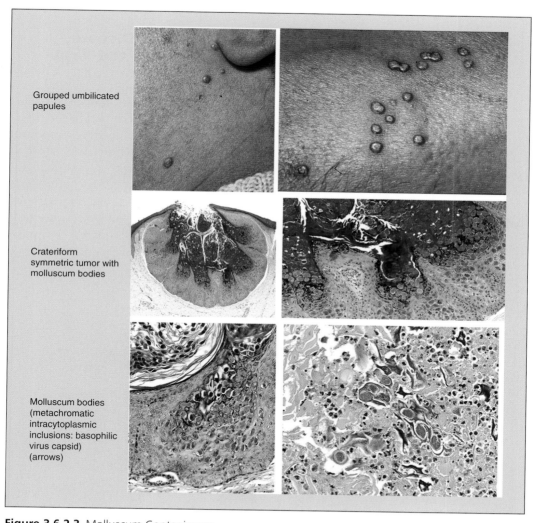

Grouped umbilicated papules

Crateriform symmetric tumor with molluscum bodies

Molluscum bodies (metachromatic intracytoplasmic inclusions: basophilic virus capsid) (arrows)

Figure 3.6.2.3 Molluscum Contagiosum.
Source: Burg et al. (2019). *Atlas of Dermatopathology: Tumors, Nevi, and Cysts* (p. 38). Oxford: Wiley.

CF: Molluscum poxvirus is the causative agent. Typically, children and immunocompromised patients are affected. Lesions are mostly multiple, inflamed, or eczematous. Characteristically, the lesions are elevated papules with a central dell.

HF:

- Exophytic symmetrical umbilicated epithelial tumor with sharp margins
- Central dell filled with necrotic keratinocytes that harbor large, basophilic intracytoplasmic inclusions (molluscum bodies); virus capsid may show immunohistochemical positivity for MelanA
- Surrounding cellular inflammatory infiltrate may mimic lymphoproliferative process due to high number of interspersed CD30-positive lymphocytes and CD123-positive plasmacytoid dendritic cells. Similar immunophenotypes may be encountered in parapox virus infection (orf)
- Flame figures may be present

DD: Verrucae planae; lepromatous leprosy.

Reference

Cribier, B., Scrivener, Y., & Grosshans, E. (2001). Molluscum contagiosum: Histologic patterns and associated lesions. A study of 578 cases. *Am J Dermatopathol*, **23**(2), 99–103.

Ishikawa, M. K., Arps, D. P., Chow, C., Hocker, T. L., & Fullen, D. R. (2015). Histopathological features of molluscum contagiosum other than molluscum bodies. *Histopathology*, **67**(6), 836–842.

Lee, S., Park, J., Kim, D., & Na, G. (2004). Flame figures in molluscum contagiosum. *Am J Dermatopathol*, **26**(5), 441–442.

3.7 Other Skin Diseases with Suspected Viral Association

Paraviral exanthems are nonspecific reactions in which viruses cannot be identified in the skin. This heterogeneous group of diseases includes asymmetrical periflexural exanthema, eruptive pseudoangiomatosis, virus-associated trichodysplasia spinulosa, Gianotti–Crosti syndrome, gloves and sock syndrome, pityriasis rosea, pityriasis lichenoides, eruptive hypomelanosis, lichen planus, systemic lupus erythematosus.

3.7.1 Asymmetric Periflexural Exanthema of Childhood

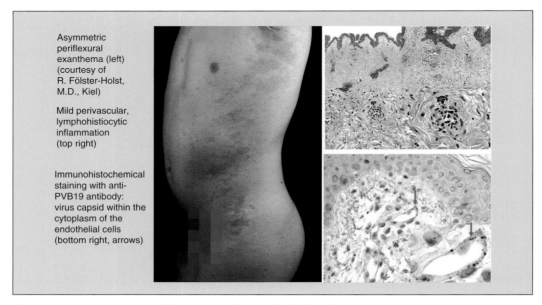

Asymmetric periflexural exanthema (left) (courtesy of R. Fölster-Holst, M.D., Kiel)

Mild perivascular, lymphohistiocytic inflammation (top right)

Immunohistochemical staining with anti-PVB19 antibody: virus capsid within the cytoplasm of the endothelial cells (bottom right, arrows)

Figure 3.7.1 Asymmetric Periflexural Exanthema of Childhood.

The disease occurs in children and in adults.

CF: Tiny papules, asymmetrically, distributed preferentially in the unilateral axillary region of one side of the trunk.

HF: Sparse perivascular, mostly lymphocytic inflammation.

DD: Pityriasis rosea; drug reaction; contact dermatitis; Gianotti–Crosti syndrome.

Reference

Santonja, C., Pielasinski, U., Polo, J., Kutzner, H., & Requena, L. (2018). Immunohistochemical demonstration of parvovirus B19 viral protein 2 in periflexural exanthema in an adult, supporting antibody-dependent enhancement as means of endothelial uptake of the virus. *Am J Dermatopathol*, **40**(2), e19–e24.

Santonja, C., Requena, L., Polo Sabau, J., & Pielasinski Rodriguez, U. (2018). Image gallery: Immunohistochemical detection of parvovirus B19 VP2 in periflexural primary infection in an adult female patient. *Br J Dermatol*, **178**(1), e65.

3.7.2 Eruptive Pseudoangiomatosis

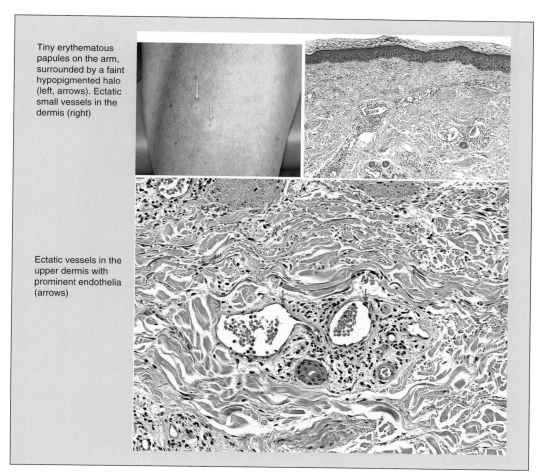

Tiny erythematous papules on the arm, surrounded by a faint hypopigmented halo (left, arrows). Ectatic small vessels in the dermis (right)

Ectatic vessels in the upper dermis with prominent endothelia (arrows)

Figure 3.7.2 Eruptive Pseudoangiomatosis.

One of the so-called paraviral exanthemas, which may be associated with echovirus or adenovirus infections.

CF: Multiple tiny erythematous annular papules, often surrounded by a faint hypopigmented halo.

HF:

- Slightly ectatic agminated vessels in the upper dermis
- Hobnail-like endothelial cells
- Sparse lymphocytic infiltrate
- No viruses detectable in the skin

DD: Other viral exanthemas; drug eruption; small plaque eruptive psoriasis; telangiectatic vascular (capillary/angiokeratoma-like) malformation; insect bite.

Reference

Chuh, A., Panzer, R., Rosenthal, A. C., Proksch, E., Kempf, W., Zawar, V., … Folster-Holst, R. (2017). Annular eruptive pseudoangiomatosis and adenovirus infection: A novel clinical variant of paraviral exanthems and a novel virus association. *Acta Derm Venereol*, **97**(3), 354–357.

Fölster-Holst, R., Zawar, V., & Chuh, A. (2017). [Paraviral exanthems]. *Hautarzt*, **68**(3), 211–216.

Neri, I., Patrizi, A., Guerrini, V., Ricci, G., & Cevenini, R. (2000). Eruptive pseudoangiomatosis. *Br J Dermatol*, **143**(2), 435–438.

Restano, L., Cavalli, R., Colonna, C., Cambiaghi, S., Alessi, E., & Caputo, R. (2005). Eruptive pseudoangiomatosis caused by an insect bite. *J Am Acad Dermatol*, **52**(1), 174–175.

3.7.3 Gianotti–Crosti Syndrome

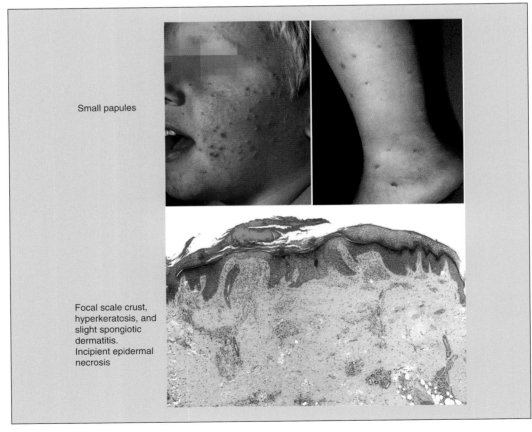

Small papules

Focal scale crust, hyperkeratosis, and slight spongiotic dermatitis. Incipient epidermal necrosis

Figure 3.7.3 Gianotti–Crosti Syndrome.
Source: Burg et al. (2015). *Atlas of Dermatopathology: Practical Differential Diagnosis by Clinicopathologic Pattern* (p. 34). Oxford: Wiley.

Suspected association with hepatitis B, coxsackievirus A-16, herpes simplex, Epstein-Barr or other virus infections.

CF: Small red papules in the face or on the limbs.

HF: Early lesions

• Spongiosis, foci of epidermal necrosis
• Exocytosis of neutrophils and eosinophils
• Intraepidermal accumulation of Langerhans cells

DD: Lichenoid dermatitis; other viral exanthemas.

Reference

Caputo, R., Gelmetti, C., Ermacora, E., Gianni, E., & Silvestri, A. (1992). Gianotti-Crosti syndrome:a retrospective analysis of 308 cases. *J Am Acad Dermatol*, **26**(2 Pt 1), 207–210.

James, W. D., Odom, R. B., & Hatch, M. H. (1982). Gianotti-Crosti-like eruption associated with coxsackievirus A-16 infection. *J Am Acad Dermatol*, **6**(5), 862–866.

Lee, S., Kim, K. Y., Hahn, C. S., Lee, M. G., & Cho, C. K. (1985). Gianotti-Crosti syndrome associated with hepatitis B surface antigen (subtype adr). *J Am Acad Dermatol*, **12**(4), 629–633.

Lowe, L., Hebert, A. A., & Duvic, M. (1989). Gianotti-Crosti syndrome associated with Epstein-Barr virus infection. *J Am Acad Dermatol*, **20**, 336–338.

Smith, K. J., & Skelton, H. (2000). Histopathologic features seen in Gianotti-Crosti syndrome secondary to Epstein-Barr virus. *J Am Acad Dermatol*, **43**(6), 1076–1079.

3.7.4 Pityriasis Lichenoides

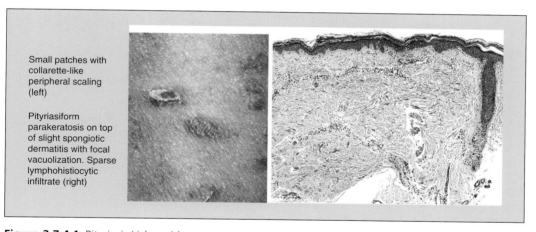

Small patches with collarette-like peripheral scaling (left)

Pityriasiform parakeratosis on top of slight spongiotic dermatitis with focal vacuolization. Sparse lymphohistiocytic infiltrate (right)

Figure 3.7.4.1 Pityriasis Lichenoides.
Source: Burg et al. (2015). *Atlas of Dermatopathology: Practical Differential Diagnosis by Clinicopathologic Pattern* (p. 32). Oxford: Wiley.

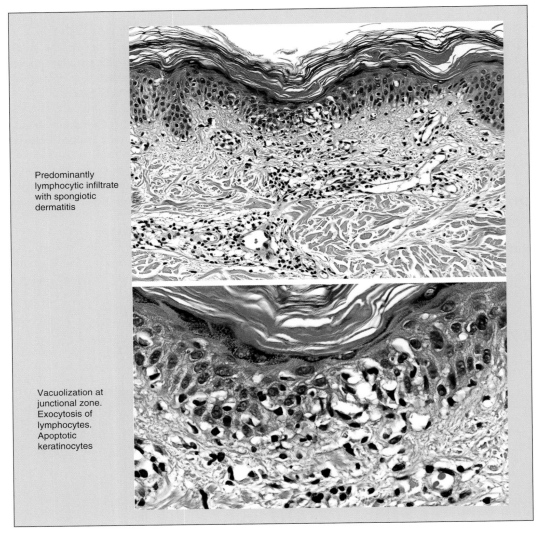

Predominantly
lymphocytic infiltrate
with spongiotic
dermatitis

Vacuolization at
junctional zone.
Exocytosis of
lymphocytes.
Apoptotic
keratinocytes

Figure 3.7.4.2 Pityriasis Lichenoides.
Source: Burg et al. (2015). *Atlas of Dermatopathology: Practical Differential Diagnosis by Clinicopathologic Pattern* (p. 33). Oxford: Wiley.

CF: Incipient pityriasis lichenoides presents with erythematous small patches or papules covered by delicate pityriasiform scales. Acute variants pityriasis lichenoides et varioliformis acuta (PLEVA) may rapidly evolve into lesions with superficial ulceration ("varioliformis"). Pityriasis lichenoides is known for its wide clinicomorphological spectrum with PLEVA and pityriasis lichenoides chronica (PLC) at either polar end and pityriasis lichenoides subacuta in the center.

HF:
- Focal pityriasiform and psoriasiform scale with neutrophils and necrotic epithelia
- Sparse acanthosis
- Apoptotic keratinocytes in variable numbers
- Interface dermatitis with vacuolization of the basal zone
- Exocytosis of mostly CD8-positive lymphocytes

- Band-like lymphocytic infiltrate in the upper dermis with interface pattern
- Remarkably, lymphomatoid papulosis type D may present with identical morphology as pityriasis lichenoides, albeit with a high number of intraepidermal CD30-positive lymphocytes
- PLEVA (acute variant of PL): Thick scale-crust with necrotic epithelia, often overlying flat erosion, with adjacent dense epidermotropic CD8-positive round cell infiltrate (interface type), and necrotic keratinocytes

DD: Drug eruption; small plaque eruptive psoriasis; lymphomatoid papulosis type D (with predominant CD30-positive epidermotropic round cells).

Reference

Benmaman, O., & Sanchez, J. L. (1988). Comparative clinicopathological study on pityriasis lichenoides chronica and small plaque parapsoriasis. *Am J Dermatopathol*, **10**(3), 189–196.

Kim, J. E., Yun, W. J., Mun, S. K., Yoon, G. S., Huh, J., Choi, J. H., & Chang, S. (2011). Pityriasis lichenoides et varioliformis acuta and pityriasis lichenoides chronica: Comparison of lesional T-cell subsets and investigation of viral associations. *J Cutan Pathol*, **38**(8), 649–656.

Nanda, A., Alshalfan, F., Al-Otaibi, M., Al-Sabah, H., & Rajy, J. M. (2013). Febrile ulceronecrotic Mucha-Habermann disease (pityriasis lichenoides et varioliformis acuta fulminans) associated with parvovirus infection. *Am J Dermatopathol*, **35**(4), 503–506.

Tomasini, D., Tomasini, C. F., Cerri, A., Sangalli, G., Palmedo, G., Hantschke, M., & Kutzner, H. (2004). Pityriasis lichenoides: A cytotoxic T-cell-mediated skin disorder. Evidence of human parvovirus B19 DNA in nine cases. *J Cutan Pathol*, **31**(8), 531–538.

Zaaroura, H., Sahar, D., Bick, T., & Bergman, R. (2018). Relationship between pityriasis lichenoides and mycosis fungoides: A clinicopathological, immunohistochemical, and molecular study. *Am J Dermatopathol*, **40**(6), 409–415.

CHAPTER 4

Parasitoses

CHAPTER MENU

4.1 Protozoan Diseases
    4.1.1 Leishmaniasis
    4.1.2 Variant: Leishmaniasis Mexicana
    4.1.3 Amebiasis: Entamoeba
          Histolytica
    4.1.4 Rhinosporidiosis

4.2 Arthropod: *Arachnids*
    4.2.1 Mites
    4.2.2 Spiders°
    4.2.3 Ticks°
    4.2.4 Insects
    4.2.5 Tungiasis (Sand Flea)

°no pictures

Atlas of Clinical Dermatopathology: Infectious and Parasitic Dermatoses, First Edition. Günter Burg,
Heinz Kutzner, Werner Kempf, Josef Feit, and Omar Sangueza.
© 2021 John Wiley & Sons Ltd. Published 2021 by John Wiley & Sons Ltd.

In parasitic infections and infestations (parasitoses), the organism, preferentially an arthropod, thrives within or on the surface (ectoparasites) of its host.

The review by Norgan and Pritt (2018), which is cited below, summarizes this complex field as follows:

«A variety of arthropods, protozoa, and helminths infect the skin and subcutaneous tissues and may be identified by anatomic pathologists in standard cytology and histology preparations. The specific organisms seen vary greatly with the patient's exposure history, including travel to or residence in endemic countries. Arthropods are the most commonly encountered parasites in the skin and subcutaneous tissues and include *Sarcoptes scabiei*, *Demodex* species, *Tunga penetrans*, and Myiasis-causing fly larvae.

Protozoal parasites such as *Leishmania* may also be common in some settings. Helminths are less often seen, and include round worms (e.g. Dirofilaria spp.), tapeworms (e.g. *Taenia solium*, *Spirometra* spp.), and flukes (e.g. *Schistosoma* spp.)".

Reference

Norgan, A. P., & Pritt, B. S. (2018). Parasitic infections of the skin and subcutaneous tissues. *Adv Anat Pathol*, **25**(2), 106–123.

Nor, N. M., & Baseri, M. M. (2015). Skin and subcutaneous infections in south-east Asia. *Curr Opin Infect Dis*, **28**(2), 133–138.

4.1 Protozoan Diseases

4.1.1 Leishmaniasis

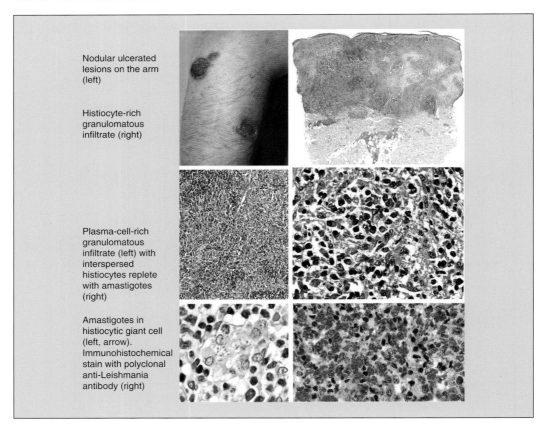

Nodular ulcerated lesions on the arm (left)

Histiocyte-rich granulomatous infiltrate (right)

Plasma-cell-rich granulomatous infiltrate (left) with interspersed histiocytes replete with amastigotes (right)

Amastigotes in histiocytic giant cell (left, arrow). Immunohistochemical stain with polyclonal anti-Leishmania antibody (right)

Figure 4.1.1.1 Leishmaniasis.

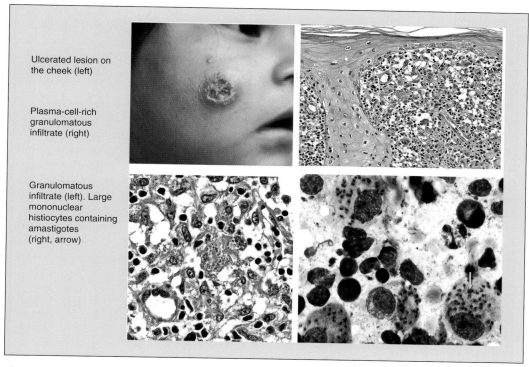

Ulcerated lesion on the cheek (left)

Plasma-cell-rich granulomatous infiltrate (right)

Granulomatous infiltrate (left). Large mononuclear histiocytes containing amastigotes (right, arrow)

Figure 4.1.1.2 Leishmaniasis.

Cutaneous leishmaniasis (CL), mucocutaneous leishmaniasis, visceral leishmaniasis (VL) or kala-azar occur by protozoan infection via female *Phlebotomus* sand flies.
CF: In cutaneous leishmaniasis, preferentially on the face, forearms, and legs, solitary or multiple crusted erythematous papules occur, which slowly evolve into open sores, exclusively at the site of previous *Phlebotomus* bites.

HF:

- Sheet-like non-caseating granuloma, "touching the epidermis" on a broad front
- Clusters of pale histiocytes, surrounded by lymphocytes and densely aggregated plasma cells
  - Amastigotes (clue: intracytoplasmic black "double dots") are preferentially found within the aggregated pale histiocytes in the center of the lesion, preferentially close to the surface
  - Flat erosions may occur
  - Advanced lesions with abundant plasma cells may resemble pseudolymphoma
  - Late lesions may be deep and present with a sarcoidal, non-caseating granuloma; plasma cells may be sparse
- Plasma cells in conjunction with clusters of pale histiocytes at subepidermal sites are a telltale sign of cutaneous leishmaniasis
- At all stages, amastigotes can be detected easily by immunohistochemical stains, preferentially at the center of the lesion, beneath the epidermis or the flat erosion
- Eosinophils
- Calcified bodies (Michaelis-Gutmann, Schaumann, psammoma, conchoidal) may be rarely found
- Anti-CD1a may be a helpful marker for some species of *Leishmania*

DD: Impetigo contagiosa; abscess; squamous cell carcinoma; various inflammatory and neoplastic disorders.

Reference

Alvarez, P., Salinas, C., & Bravo, F. (2011). Calcified bodies in New World cutaneous leishmaniasis. *Am J Dermatopathol*, **33**(8), 827–830.

Dias-Polak, D., Geffen, Y., Ben-Izhak, O., & Bergman, R. (2017). The role of histopathology and immunohistochemistry in the diagnosis of cutaneous leishmaniasis without "discernible" Leishman-Donovan bodies. *Am J Dermatopathol*, **39**(12), 890–895.

Ferrufino-Schmidt, M. C., Bravo, F., Valencia, B. M., Llanos-Cuentas, A., Boggild, A. K., & LeBoit, P. E. (2019). Is CD1a useful for leishmaniasis diagnosis in the New World? *J Cutan Pathol*, **46**(1), 90–92.

Quintella, L. P., Cuzzi, T., de Fatima Madeira, M., Valete-Rosalino, C. M., de Matos Salgueiro, M., de Camargo Ferreira e Vasconcellos, E., ... de Oliveira Schubach, A. (2011). Cutaneous leishmaniasis with pseudoepitheliomatous hyperplasia simulating squamous cell carcinoma. *Am J Dermatopathol*, **33**(6), 642–644.

Saab, J., Fedda, F., Khattab, R., Yahya, L., Loya, A., Satti, M., ... Khalifeh, I. (2012). Cutaneous leishmaniasis mimicking inflammatory and neoplastic processes: A clinical, histopathological and molecular study of 57 cases. *J Cutan Pathol*, **39**(2), 251–262.

Thilakarathne, I. K., Ratnayake, P., Vithanage, A., & Sugathadasa, D. P. (2019). Role of histopathology in the diagnosis of cutaneous leishmaniasis: A case-control study in Sri Lanka. *Am J Dermatopathol*, **41**(8), 566–570.

4.1.2 Variant: Leishmaniasis Mexicana

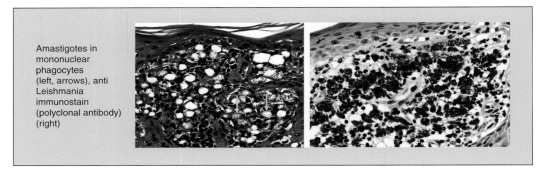

Amastigotes in mononuclear phagocytes (left, arrows), anti Leishmania immunostain (polyclonal antibody) (right)

Figure 4.1.2 Variant: Leishmaniasis Mexicana.

Leishmania mexicana, like all *Leishmania* spp., is an obligate intracellular protozoan parasite which is endemic to Mexico and Central America. Clinical and histologic features are identical with other forms of cutaneous leishmaniasis. Differentiation is feasible by molecular methods (PCR/sequencing).

Reference

Grimaldi, G., Jr., Moriearty, P. L., & Hoff, R. (1980). Leishmania mexicana: Immunology and histopathology in C3H mice. *Exp Parasitol*, **50**(1), 45–56.

Andrade-Narvaez, F. J., Medina-Peralta, S., Vargas-Gonzalez, A., Canto-Lara, S. B., & Estrada-Parra, S. (2005). The histopathology of cutaneous leishmaniasis due to Leishmania (Leishmania) mexicana in the Yucatan peninsula, Mexico. *Rev Inst Med Trop Sao Paulo*, **47**(4), 191–194.

4.1.3 Amebiasis: Entamoeba Histolytica

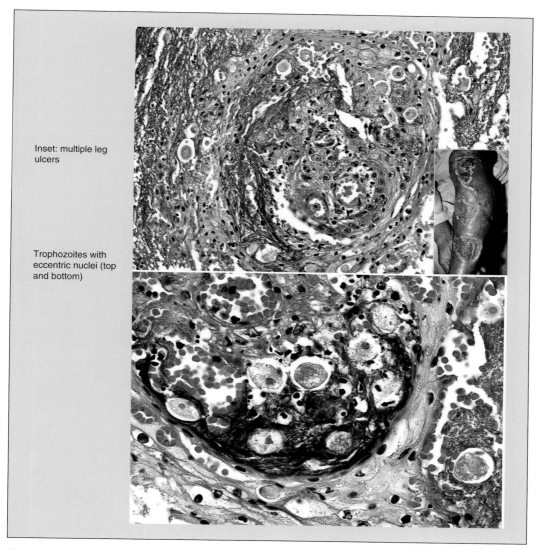

Inset: multiple leg ulcers

Trophozoites with eccentric nuclei (top and bottom)

Figure 4.1.3 Amebiasis: Entamoeba Histolytica.

Amebiasis primarily occurs in tropical and subtropical areas; rarely in Europe. Gastrointestinal infection is caused by *Entamoeba histolytica*. The skin may get affected via primary infection or more frequently by per continuitatem extension of rectal amebiasis to the anus, perianal skin, and vulva, or via liver abscess perforating to the abdominal wall. Acanthamebiasis (e.g. via contaminated contact lenses) may cause keratitis, followed by CNS involvement.
CF: Nodular and cystic lesions, which evolve into deep ulcers with undermined and elevated borders.

HF:

- Pseudocarcinomatous (pseudoepitheliomatous) hyperplasia of the spongiotic epidermis with liquefactive necrosis, bordering shallow ulceration
- Hematophagous trophozoites (erythrophagocytosis) in the dermis, showing clear cytoplasm and an eccentric nucleus. (Clue: ganglion-cell like organisms)
- Admixed granulomatous or suppurative infiltrate

DD: Abscess; cysts; tropical ulcer.

Reference

Magana, M., Magana, M. L., Alcantara, A., & Perez-Martin, M. A. (2004). Histopathology of cutaneous amebiasis. *Am J Dermatopathol*, **26**(4), 280–284.

Ramdial, P. K., Calonje, E., Singh, B., Bagratee, J. S., Singh, S. M., & Sydney, C. (2007). Amebiasis cutis revisited. *J Cutan Pathol*, **34**(8), 620–628.

4.1.4 Rhinosporidiosis

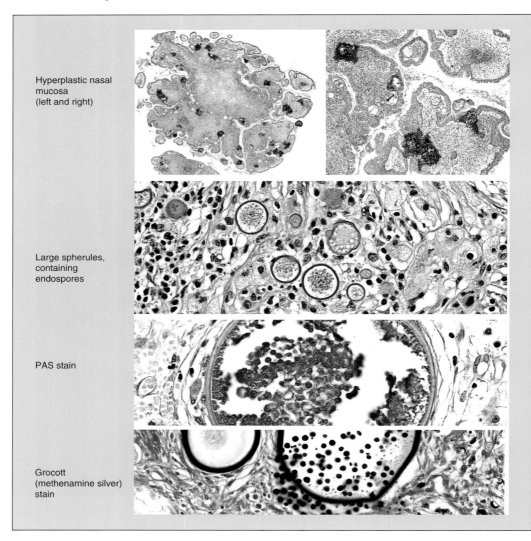

Hyperplastic nasal mucosa (left and right)

Large spherules, containing endospores

PAS stain

Grocott (methenamine silver) stain

Figure 4.1.4 Rhinosporidiosis.

Rhinosporidium seeberi, the causative agent of rhinosporidiosis, is an aquatic proto-zoon, morphologically mimicking a fungus. Preferential sites of infection are the nasal or ocular mucosa. Males in tropical areas are more often infected than females. **CF**: The cornified skin is only rarely affected. Mucosal surfaces are primarily involved. Papules and large strawberry-like polyps occur on the nasal, ocular, and nasopharyngeal mucosa.

HF:

- Polypoid exophytic mass
- Presence of sporangia (large spherules, replete with small round "endospores") in the submucosal propria (Grocott and PAS)
- Mixed accompanying round cell infiltrate with histiocytes, neutrophils, lymphocytes and plasma cells, and few giant cells in the adjacent propria
- No cellular atypia (versus lethal midline granuloma [NK/T-cell lymphoma] with marked pleomorphism)

DD: Lethal midline granuloma (NK/T-cell lymphoma); cryptococcosis.

Reference

de Silva, N. R., Huegel, H., Atapattu, D. N., Arseculeratne, S. N., Kumarasiri, R., Gunawardena, S., ... Fernando, R. (2001). Cell-mediated immune responses (CMIR) in human rhinosporidiosis. *Mycopathologia*, **152**(2), 59–68.

Sudarshan, V., Gahine, R., Daharwal, A., Kujur, P., Hussain, N., Krishnani, C., & Tiwari, S. K. (2012). Rhinosporidiosis of the parotid duct presenting as a parotid duct cyst – a report of three cases. *Indian J Med Microbiol*, **30**(1), 108–111.

4.2 Arthropod: *Arachnids*

4.2.1 Mites

There is a large variety of different mites, and apart from scabies and harvest mites, include *Cheyletiella* mites, poultry mites, house dust mites, and other species.

4.2.1.1 Demodex Folliculorum

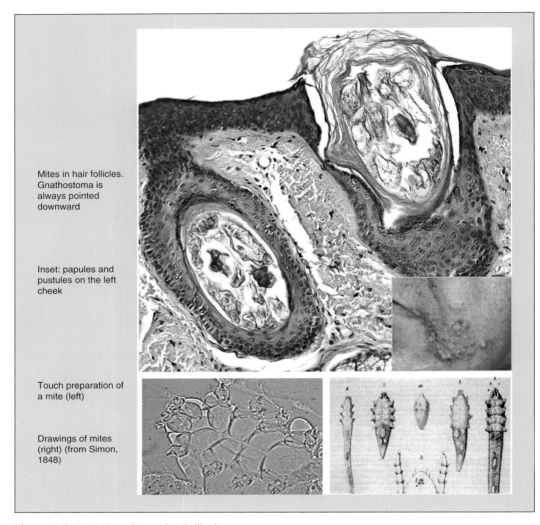

Mites in hair follicles. Gnathostoma is always pointed downward

Inset: papules and pustules on the left cheek

Touch preparation of a mite (left)

Drawings of mites (right) (from Simon, 1848)

Figure 4.2.1.1 Mites: Demodex Folliculorum.

CF: *Demodex folliculorum* mites thrive within hair follicles, induce acute folliculitis, and present as papules and pustules, typically mimicking rosacea.

HF:

- Dilated follicle ostia
- Follicles containing keratotic debris and mites, single or in groups
- Heads of mites (*Gnathostoma*) typically directed downward towards the hair bulb
- Mononuclear and neutrophilic infiltrates around and in the involved follicle
- Perifollicular granulomatous infiltrate (late)

DD: Rosacea; perioral dermatitis; seborrheic dermatitis.

Reference

Helou, W., Avitan-Hersh, E., & Bergman, R. (2016). Demodex folliculitis of the scalp: clinicopathological study of an uncommon entity. *Am J Dermatopathol*, **38**(9), 658–663.

4.2.1.2 Scabies

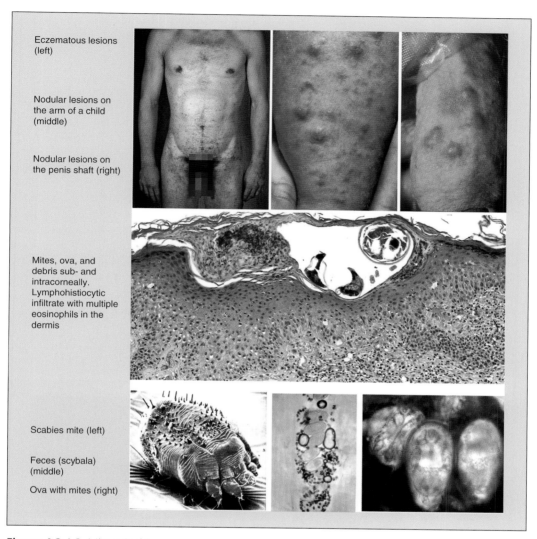

Eczematous lesions (left)

Nodular lesions on the arm of a child (middle)

Nodular lesions on the penis shaft (right)

Mites, ova, and debris sub- and intracorneally. Lymphohistiocytic infiltrate with multiple eosinophils in the dermis

Scabies mite (left)

Feces (scybala) (middle)

Ova with mites (right)

Figure 4.2.1.2 Mites: Scabies.

This is an ectoparasitic infection by the mite *Sarcoptes scabiei* var. *hominis*. Transmission is via direct body contact or contact with garments infested with mites or eggs. The male mite dies after mating while the female is tunneling through the stratum corneum, laying eggs, and depositing brownish feces (scybala).

CF: Pruritic eczematous papules and excoriations, preferentially at the interdigital sites, on the wrists and on the penis. In young children, palms and soles may also be affected. Feces and proteinaceous deposits of the mites may cause additional pruritic allergic eczematous reactions. Scratching-induced bacterial superinfection may evolve into severe impetiginization.

Variants: Crusted ("Norwegian") scabies; nodular scabies (mimicking pseudolymphoma).

HF:

- Acanthosis with exocytosis and spongiosis
- Dermoscopy reveals intracorneal tunnels with mites at the end of the tunnel
- Step sections show intracorneal or subcorneal burrows with mites, eggs, and brownish feces (scybala)
- Perivascular lymphocytic infiltrate with eosinophils and few plasma cells
- Scabies granuloma (late): Nodular pseudolymphomatous infiltrates with many CD30-positive cells may mimic lymphomatoid papulosis or pseudolymphoma
- Crusted ("Norwegian") scabies: Thick, layered hyperkeratosis containing a plethora of mites
- Polariscopic examination (birefringence) may be a helpful clue for the visualization of mites and scybala

DD: Langerhans cell histiocytosis; CD30-positive lymphoma; lymphomatoid papulosis; pseudolymphomas.

Reference

Bhattacharjee, P., & Glusac, E. J. (2007). Langerhans cell hyperplasia in scabies: A mimic of Langerhans cell histiocytosis. *J Cutan Pathol*, **34**(9), 716–720.

Foo, C. W., Florell, S. R., & Bowen, A. R. (2013). Polarizable elements in scabies infestation: A clue to diagnosis. *J Cutan Pathol*, **40**(1), 6–10.

Gallardo, F., Barranco, C., Toll, A., & Pujol, R. M. (2002). CD30 antigen expression in cutaneous inflammatory infiltrates of scabies: A dynamic immunophenotypic pattern that should be distinguished from lymphomatoid papulosis. *J Cutan Pathol*, **29**(6), 368–373.

4.2.1.3 Variant: Scabies Crustosa

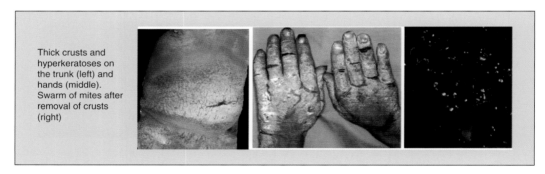

Thick crusts and hyperkeratoses on the trunk (left) and hands (middle). Swarm of mites after removal of crusts (right)

Figure 4.2.1.3 Variant: Scabies Crustosa.

Crusted scabies is a rare variant of scabies, occurring preferentially in immunocompromised people. The suffix "Norwegica," which traditionally has been used, is a misnomer: this variant of scabies does not have any Scandinavian ties at all.

CF: Massive hyperkeratotic crusts are found preferentially on the extremities, on the face and capillitium. The crusts are highly contagious, as they are replete with myriads of mites.

HF: Massive hyperkeratotic scales with a plethora of scabies mites, ovula, and scybala.

DD: Other hyperkeratotic disorders, psoriasis vulgaris, tylotic eczema.

4.2.1.4 Trombidiosis (Harvest Mites; Chigger Itch)

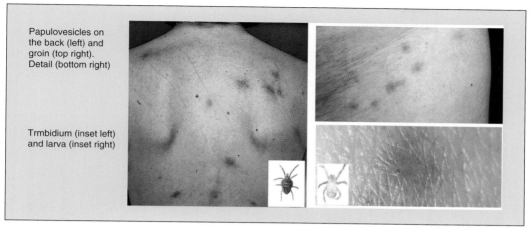

Papulovesicles on the back (left) and groin (top right). Detail (bottom right)

Trmbidium (inset left) and larva (inset right)

Figure 4.2.1.4 Trombidiosis (Harvest Mites; Chigger Itch).

In the fall (in Europe), the larva of *Trombicula autumnalis*, which may temporarily attach to the skin and suck blood, causes pruritic allergic reactions mostly in people who have been in the outdoors.

CF: Small itchy macules appear preferentially at the rims of tight clothing (socks, underwear, belt), which evolve into tiny papulovesicles. Excoriation and bacterial superinfection may result from vigorous scratching.

HF:

• Slight superficial erosion or spongiosis only
• Moderate lymphocytic infiltrate in the dermis with eosinophils
• Mites not present

DD: All other arthropod bite reactions.

4.2.2 Spiders°

CF: Painful erythema followed by urticarial or papular induration and central hemorrhagic necrosis at the site of previous spider bite. Systemic symptoms (pain, fever) may

occur. Spider bites also may be a possible trigger for acute generalized exanthematous pustulosis (AGEP).

HF:

• Necrosis at the site of spider bite
• Hemorrhage and accompanying vasculopathy (thrombi)
• Polymorphous dermal infiltrate, consisting of lymphocytes, neutrophils, eosinophils

DD: Pyoderma gangrenosum; pyogenic granuloma; vasculitis; trauma; thrombotic or embolic infarction.

Reference

Davidovici, B. B., Pavel, D., Cagnano, E., Rozenman, D., Halevy, S., EuroScar, & Regi, S. s. g. (2006). Acute generalized exanthematous pustulosis following a spider bite: Report of 3 cases. *J Am Acad Dermatol,* **55**(3), 525–529.

Elston, D. M., Eggers, J. S., Schmidt, W. E., Storrow, A. B., Doe, R. H., McGlasson, D., & Fischer, J. R. (2000). Histological findings after brown recluse spider envenomation. *Am J Dermatopathol,* **22**(3), 242–246.

4.2.3 Ticks°

Ticks may serve as vectors for bacterial (*Borrelia*, *Ehrlichia*) or viral organisms. Sometimes chitinous remnants of the tick's head (hypostome) can be detected clinically or histologically in the center of the lesion. There is a dense superficial and deep mixed infiltrate, containing many eosinophils, followed by granulomatous changes (late). Vasculopathy is not unusual (early).

4.2.4 Insects

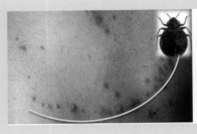 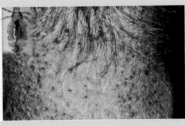

Quasi regular curved traces of *Cimex* bites (left). Inset: *Cimex lectularius*

"Dirty" irregular eczematous lesions on the neck (right). Inset: *Pediculus capitis*

Figure 4.2.4 Arthropods: Insects Cimex Lectularius; Bedbugs (left). Pediculosis Capitis (right).

A variety of insects may be involved in cutaneous infestations, mosquito bites being the most common ones. Clinical inspection and demonstration of the ectoparasites and their eggs or larvae is diagnostic in most cases. The group of clinically relevant insects includes bedbugs (*Cimex lectularius*), various types of pediculi, fly larvae (myiasis), which grow within the dermis, and may also be found on open wounds.

CF: The cutaneous reactions range from simple pruritic erythema to bluish, hemorrhagic macular lesions, papules, longstanding wheals, and strong hemorrhagic bullous reactions with necrosis. Exaggerated insect bite reactions may be seen in hyperergic individuals or patients with leukemia/lymphoma or positive for HIV. They are at a particular risk of developing massive arthropod bite reaction (e.g. classic "mosquito-bite-reaction").

HF:

- Spongiosis and exocytosis

- Subepidermal edema, occasionally evolving into subepidermal bulla
- Bullous reactions may show hemorrhage
- Superficial and deep, wedge-shaped lymphocytic infiltrate with eosinophils
- Neutrophils en masse, particularly in lesions induced by lice
- Eosinophils in the dermis, occasionally invading the epidermis, are a strong diagnostic hint
- Vasculopathy or secondary leukocytoclastic vasculitis may occur

DD: All parasitoses; mantle cell lymphoma; eruptive pseudoangiomatosis.

Reference

Haddad, V., Jr., Cardoso, J. L., Lupi, O., & Tyring, S. K. (2012). Tropical dermatology: Venomous arthropods and human skin: Part I. Insecta. *J Am Acad Dermatol*, **67**(3), 331.

Khamaysi, Z., Dodiuk-Gad, R. P., Weltfriend, S., Ben-Arieh, Y., Dann, E. J., Sahar, D., & Bergman, R. (2005). Insect bite-like reaction associated with mantle cell lymphoma: Clinicopathological, immunopathological, and molecular studies. *Am J Dermatopathol*, **27**(4), 290–295.

Smith, K. J., Skelton, H. G., 3rd, Vogel, P., Yeager, J., Baxter, D., & Wagner, K. F. (1993).

Exaggerated insect bite reactions in patients positive for HIV. Military Medical Consortium for the Advancement of Retroviral Research. *J Am Acad Dermatol*, **29**(2 Pt 1), 269–272.

4.2.5 Tungiasis (Sand Flea)

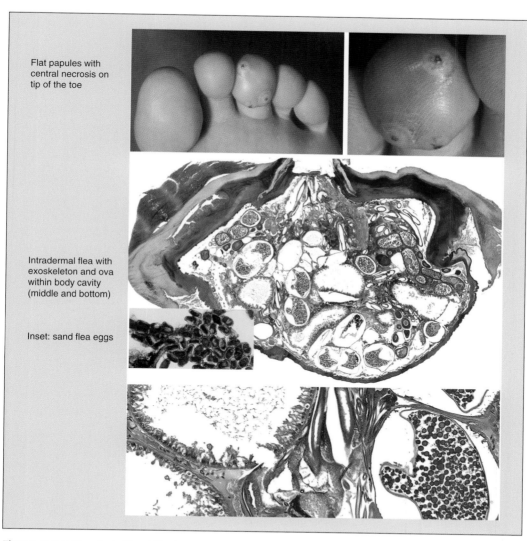

Flat papules with central necrosis on tip of the toe

Intradermal flea with exoskeleton and ova within body cavity (middle and bottom)

Inset: sand flea eggs

Figure 4.2.5 Tungiasis (Sand Flea).

The female sand flea (Tunga penetrans) thrives in the skin, where it produces several hundred eggs.

CF: In tropical climates, small pruritic centrally ulcerated papules or nodules preferentially occur on the toes, under the toenails, and at interdigital sites.

HF: Intradermally located female flea, bearing hundreds of eggs within its body. Accompanying polymorphous round cell infiltrate.

DD: Subungual warts; pyogenic granuloma.

Reference

Coates, S. J., Thomas, C., Chosidow, O., Engelman, D., & Chang, A. Y. (2020). Part II – Ectoparasites: Pediculosis and tungiasis. *J Am Acad Dermatol*, **82**(3), 551–569.

Nazzaro, G., Genovese, G., & Veraldi, S. (2019). Clinical and histopathologic study of 39 patients with imported tungiasis. *J Cutan Pathol*, **46**(4), 251–255.

CHAPTER 5
Helminthic Infections (Parasitic Worms)

CHAPTER MENU

5.1 Larva Migrans (Plumber's Itch; Creeping Eruption)
5.2 Filariasis
5.3 Onchocerciasis (River Blindness)
5.4 Cysticercosis
5.5 Sparganosis

5.6 Schistosomiasis (Bilharziasis)
5.7 Cercarial Dermatitis (Swimmer's Itch)
5.8 Annelida (Ringed Worms; Segmented Worms)°
5.9 Hirudinea (Leeches)

°no pictures

Atlas of Clinical Dermatopathology: Infectious and Parasitic Dermatoses, First Edition. Günter Burg,
Heinz Kutzner, Werner Kempf, Josef Feit, and Omar Sangueza.
© 2021 John Wiley & Sons Ltd. Published 2021 by John Wiley & Sons Ltd.

Helminths are macroparasites, usually affecting the intestinal tract, the lymph, or blood vessels, and occasionally the skin. Humans are infected by eggs or larvae, which are either ingested, transmitted by bite of an insect, which serves as vector – or by direct penetration into the skin. There is no consistent taxonomy of helminths. The main groups comprise roundworms (nematodes), tapeworms (cestodes), and flukes (trematodes).

5.1 Larva Migrans (Plumber's Itch; Creeping Eruption)

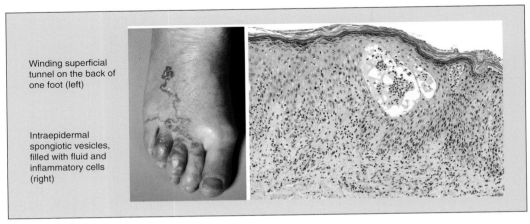

Winding superficial tunnel on the back of one foot (left)

Intraepidermal spongiotic vesicles, filled with fluid and inflammatory cells (right)

Figure 5.1 Larva Migrans (Plumber's Itch; Creeping Eruption).

In tropical and subtropical countries, larvae of various nematodes of the hookworm family, most commonly *Ancylostoma braziliense*, which is present in animal feces and in the soil, cause cutaneous "creeping eruption." Larva currens that is caused by the roundworm *Strongyloides stercoralis* presents with rapidly progressing migratory paths in the skin.

CF: Slightly elevated pruritic erythematous winding path, preferentially on the feet and the buttocks. The jagged and characteristically winding erythematous path is highly characteristic and pathognomonic of larva migrans.

HF: Intraepidermal spongiotic vesicles, left by the slowly migrating larva. In cutaneous biopsies, larvae are seldom demonstrated as they migrate up to few millimeters ahead of the clinically visible tunnel. Accompanying dermal edema with inflammatory lymphocytic infiltrate and many eosinophils.

DD: Other creeping eruptions; cutaneous cryptococcosis; loiasis.

Reference

Lockmann, A., Seitz, C. S., Schon, M. P., & Mossner, R. (2018). Creeping eruption and eosinophilic folliculitis: Atypical cutaneous larva migrans. *J Dtsch Dermatol Ges*, **16**(2), 202–204.

Ma, D. L., & Vano-Galvan, S. (2016). IMAGES IN CLINICAL MEDICINE. Creeping eruption – Cutaneous larva migrans. *N Engl J Med*, **374**(14), e16.

Vanhaecke, C., Perignon, A., Monsel, G., Regnier, S., Paris, L., & Caumes, E. (2014). Aetiologies of creeping eruption: 78 cases. *Br J Dermatol*, **170**(5), 1166–1169.

5.2 Filariasis

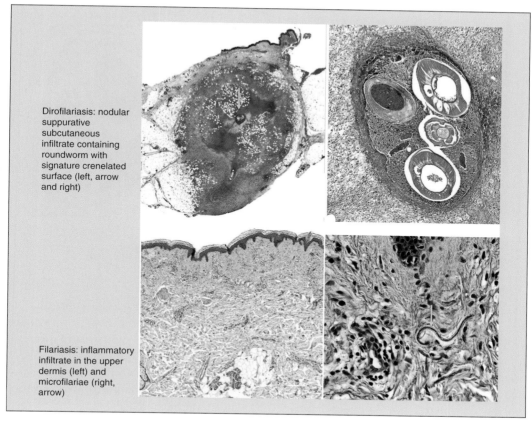

Dirofilariasis: nodular suppurative subcutaneous infiltrate containing roundworm with signature crenelated surface (left, arrow and right)

Filariasis: inflammatory infiltrate in the upper dermis (left) and microfilariae (right, arrow)

Figure 5.2 Filariasis.

Culex or *Aedes* mosquitoes serve as vectors for human roundworm infection. Subcutaneous filariasis is caused by *Loa loa* (eye worm). In classic filariasis, humans are the only host. The adult female filaria of the *Wuchereria bancrofti* species within lymph nodes release microfilaria into the blood stream. In particular, they cause obstruction of lymph vessels that eventually results in massive lymphedema (elephantiasis).

CF: Apart from potentially severe extracutaneous symptoms, obstruction of the lymph vessels leads to massive edematous swelling (elephantiasis) and subsequent fibrosis, preferentially on the legs and the scrotum.

HF: Edematous and fibrotic thickening of the skin with dilated lymph vessels. Dense lymphocytic inflammatory reaction with many eosinophils. In advanced stages, edema gradually resolves and is replaced by fibrosis.

DD: Lymphedema caused by metastatic obstruction of lymph vessels; lymphangiosarcoma.

Reference

Krishnamoorthy, N., Viswanathan, S., Rekhi, B., & Jambhekar, N. A. (2012). Lymphangiosarcoma arising after 33 years within a background of chronic filariasis: A case report with review of literature. *J Cutan Pathol*, **39**(1), 52–55.

Wiwanitkit, V. (2012). Lymphangiosarcoma and filariasis. *J Cutan Pathol*, **39**(8), 813.

5.3 Onchocerciasis (River Blindness)

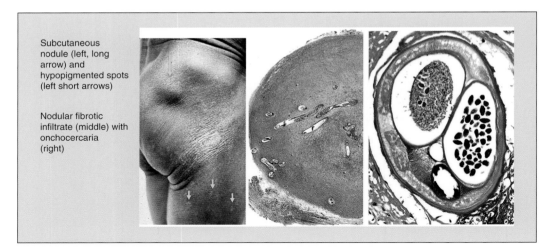

Subcutaneous nodule (left, long arrow) and hypopigmented spots (left short arrows)

Nodular fibrotic infiltrate (middle) with onchocercaria (right)

Figure 5.3 Onchocerciasis.

In endemic areas of Africa and Central America, the black fly (buffalo gnat) is the vector for *Onchocerca volvulus*. Subsequent to the bite of a fly, larvae develop and migrate via blood vessels into the subcutaneous tissue, where they mature into adult worms, the microfilaria. In endemic areas, onchocerciasis is one of the most frequent causes of ("river") blindness.

CF: Subcutaneous nodules replete with organisms, itching onchocercal dermatitis, lichenoid plaques, spotted depigmentation ("leopard skin"), and accompanying blindness are the leading clinical symptoms.

HF:

- Multitude of entangled worms of both sexes (paired worms) within encapsulated nodules (onchocercoma)
- Microfilaria in the papillary dermis
- Subepidermal edema and strong inflammatory response with formation of microabscesses around necrotic larvae
- Mixed cellular infiltrate, with histiocytes, lymphocytes, neutrophils, eosinophils, and plasma cells

DD: Filarial lymphedema; other worms; mycobacterial or fungal infections; lipoma.

Reference

Lai, J. H., Walsh, N. M., Pritt, B. S., Sloan, L., Gibson, L. E., Desormeau, L., & Haldane, D. J. (2014). Cutaneous manifestations of a zoonotic Onchocerca species in an adult male, acquired in Nova Scotia, Canada. *J Clin Microbiol*, **52**(5), 1768–1770.

5.4 Cysticercosis

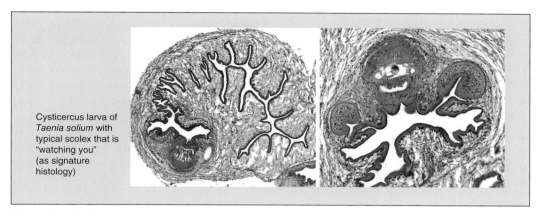

Cysticercus larva of *Taenia solium* with typical scolex that is "watching you" (as signature histology)

Figure 5.4 Cysticercosis.

Infection occurs via fecal-oral spread: ingestion of the tapeworm eggs that are shed with the feces of humans harboring adult *Taenia solium*. Humans are the intermediate host for the larvae, which may migrate to the brain and cause neurological symptoms (seizures). Infiltration into other organs (heart, eyes), including the skin, is not uncommon.

CF: Swelling and subcutaneous painful lumps with cysts, mostly on the trunk and the limbs. There often are characteristic accompanying neurological symptoms (seizures).

HF: Larva with typical scolex.

DD: Lipoma; subcutaneous cyst; pseudotumor.

Reference

Ponnighaus, J. M., Nkhosa, P., & Baum, H. P. (2001). [Cutaneous manifestation of cysticercosis]. *Hautarzt*, **52**(12), 1098–1100.

5.5 Sparganosis

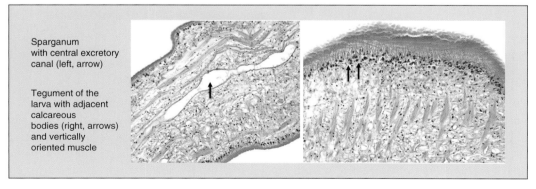

Sparganum with central excretory canal (left, arrow)

Tegument of the larva with adjacent calcareous bodies (right, arrows) and vertically oriented muscle

Figure 5.5 Sparganosis.

Ingestion of contaminated water (cyclops, "water fleas") or contact with an intermediate host can lead to infection where humans are the second intermediate host of the tapeworm larva (sparganum).

CF: Swelling with subcutaneous nodule.

HF: Free-floating larva (sparganum) within a wide, non-encapsulated cavity. The sparganum shows a typical central canal, surrounded by multiple basophilic calcareous bodies, small muscles bundles, and a crenelated tegument.

DD: Lipoma.

Reference

Chang, J. H., Lin, O. S., & Yeh, K. T. (1999). Subcutaneous sparganosis – a case report and a review of human sparganosis in Taiwan. *Kaohsiung J Med Sci*, **15**(9), 567–571.

Etges, F. J., & Marinakis, V. (1991). Formation and excretion of calcareous bodies by the metacestode (Tetrathyridium) of Mesocestoides vogae. *J Parasitol*, **77**(4), 595–602.

Sarukawa, S., Kawanabe, T., Yagasaki, A., Shimizu, A., & Shimada, S. (2007). Case of subcutaneous sparganosis: Use of imaging in definitive preoperative diagnosis. *J Dermatol*, **34**(9), 654–657.

5.6 Schistosomiasis (Bilharziasis)

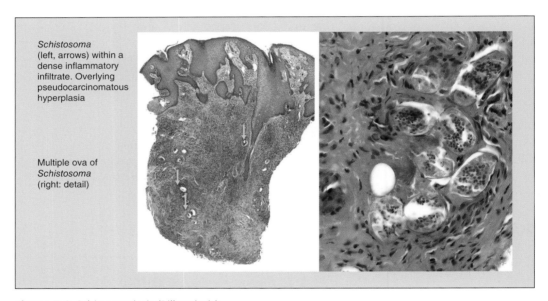

Schistosoma (left, arrows) within a dense inflammatory infiltrate. Overlying pseudocarcinomatous hyperplasia

Multiple ova of Schistosoma (right: detail)

Figure 5.6 Schistosomiasis (Bilharziasis).

The endemic infection is caused by various species of the superfamily Schistosomatoidea. The most common species that cause infection in humans are *S. haematobium, S. japonicum,* and *S. mansoni*.

Life cycle of the *Schistosoma* species: Infested human urine or human feces, which is shed into shallow bodies of water, are the primary sources of *Schistosoma* eggs. In the water, these eggs develop into miracidia, which enter the bodies of snails, where they mature. They finally leave their snail hosts as fork-tailed cercariae. Finally, waterborne cercariae enter the human body via the skin (legs). In the human host, cercariae migrate via veins and lymphatic system to the splanchnic and urogenital venous plexus, where they mature into adult worms.

Migration of parasites to the skin into preexisting pathologic conditions may occur (bilharziasis cutanea tarda).

CF: Pruritic papular dermatitis, preferentially on the legs (early), followed by allergic febrile reaction with accompanying urticaria, edema, arthritis, eosinophilia (intermediate stage). Chronic stage with involvement of internal organs (lungs, liver, bladder, CNS). In the skin, often intensive inflammation with verrucous papules and nodules, preferentially at perineal and gluteal sites. These inflamed skin lesions may contain *Schistosoma* eggs, albeit in very low numbers.

HF: Eggs are rarely found in chronic skin lesions. Leading histopathological changes are dense infiltrates mainly composed of neutrophils and eosinophils. In routine sections, cercariae can be found in exceptionally rare cases.

DD: Arthropod bites; urticaria; other worm infections.

Reference

Davis-Reed, L., & Theis, J. H. (2000). Cutaneous schistosomiasis: Report of a case and review of the literature. *J Am Acad Dermatol*, **42**(4), 678–680.

Eulderink, F., Gryseels, B., van Kampen, W. J., & de Regt, J. (1994). Haematobium schistosomiasis presenting in the Netherlands as a skin disease. *Am J Dermatopathol*, **16**(4), 434–438.

Matz, H., Berger, S., Gat, A., & Brenner, S. (2003). Bilharziasis cutanea tarda: A rare presentation of schistosomiasis. *J Am Acad Dermatol*, **49**(5), 961–962.

5.7 Cercarial Dermatitis (Swimmer's Itch)

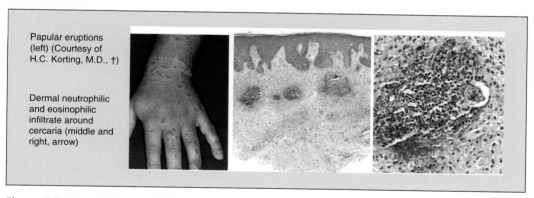

Papular eruptions (left) (Courtesy of H.C. Korting, M.D., †)

Dermal neutrophilic and eosinophilic infiltrate around cercaria (middle and right, arrow)

Figure 5.7 Cercarial Dermatitis (Swimmer's Itch).

Fresh water fowl (ducks) are the primary hosts of schistosomes of the *Trichobilharzia* genus. Infected ducks release cercariae into the water, where they usually infect snails (complete life cycle). Instead, bathing humans may get infected per chance, albeit only very superficially, with cercariae not being able to pass through the human skin (incomplete life cycle). At the site of infection, intensely pruritic urticarial erythema develop (swimmer's itch).

CF: Macular and papular intensely pruritic and urticarial lesions, preferentially at water-exposed body sites.

HF: Only in exceptional cases, cercariae may be encountered in the subepidermal dermis, surrounded by perivascular eosinophilic infiltrate.

DD: Irritant or allergic contact dermatitis.

Reference

Soldanova, M., Selbach, C., Kalbe, M., Kostadinova, A., & Sures, B. (2013). Swimmer's itch: Etiology, impact, and risk factors in Europe. *Trends Parasitol*, **29**(2), 65–74.

5.9 Hirudinea (Leeches)

5.8 Annelida (Ringed Worms; Segmented Worms)°

They are ectoparasites and do not belong to the helminths sensu stricto. Helminths are endoparasites, thriving in the gut, in the lymph and blood vessels. The term "ringworm" ("taenia," "tinea") is misleading as it traditionally designates fungal infections (dermatophytosis).

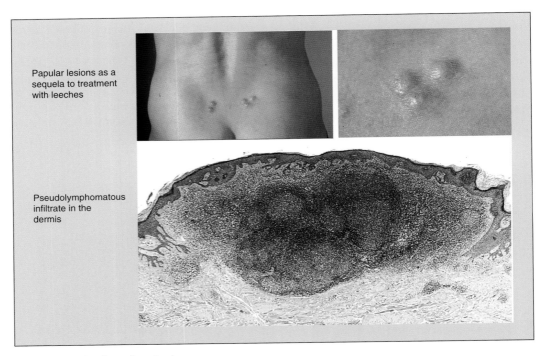

Papular lesions as a sequela to treatment with leeches

Pseudolymphomatous infiltrate in the dermis

Figure 5.9 Hirudinea (Leeches).

Hematophageous leeches of the species *Hirudo medicinalis* are ectoparasites and are not classified as helminths, which are endoparasites. Traditionally they have been applied in medicine for a variety of indications. With their sharp teeth, they attach to their host, and while sucking blood, they release anticoagulant and anesthetic saliva into the host. Cross-infection with the gram-negative bacterium *Aeromonas hydrophila*, which is present in the mouth and the gut of the worm, must be considered when working with *Hirudo medicinalis*.

HF: Remarkably cellular pseudolymphomatous infiltrate, occasionally with germinal centers, with eosinophils and plasma cells.

DD: Characteristic erythematous maculopapular and nodular lesions at the sites of previous leech bites.

Reference

Khelifa, E., Kaya, G., & Laffitte, E. (2013). Cutaneous pseudolymphomas after leech therapy. *J Dermatol*, **40**(8), 674–675.

Beer, A.-M., Fey, S., Kuhnen, C., & Mentzel, T. (2001). Kutane Arthropodenreaktion nach Blutegeltherapie. *Akt Dermatol*, **27**, 42–46.

CHAPTER 6

Sepsis

CHAPTER MENU

6.1 Septic Vasculitis
6.2 Bacterial Sepsis
    6.2.1 Gonococcal Sepsis

6.3 Fungal Sepsis
    6.3.1 Variant: Penicillium Marinum Sepsis
    6.3.2 Variant: Candida Sepsis
    6.3.3 Variant: Aspergillus Sepsis

Atlas of Clinical Dermatopathology: Infectious and Parasitic Dermatoses, First Edition. Günter Burg,
Heinz Kutzner, Werner Kempf, Josef Feit, and Omar Sangueza.
© 2021 John Wiley & Sons Ltd. Published 2021 by John Wiley & Sons Ltd.

6.1 Septic Vasculitis

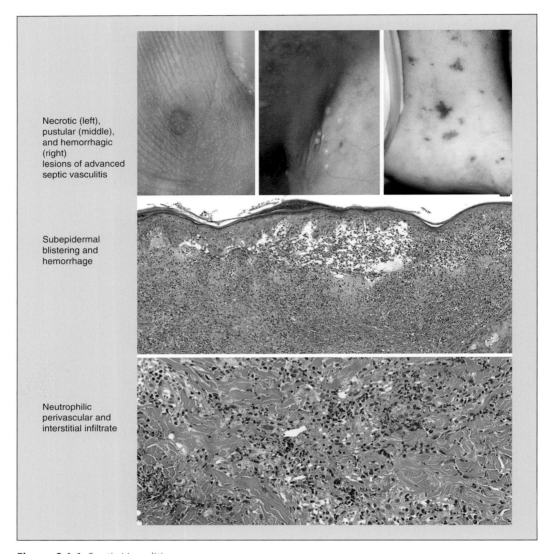

Necrotic (left), pustular (middle), and hemorrhagic (right) lesions of advanced septic vasculitis

Subepidermal blistering and hemorrhage

Neutrophilic perivascular and interstitial infiltrate

Figure 6.1.1 Septic Vasculitis.

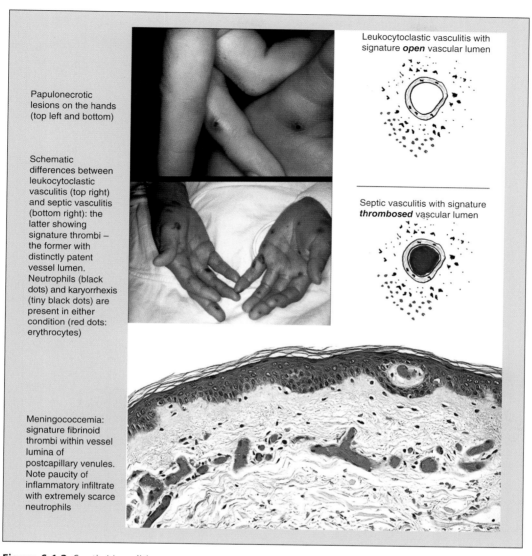

Papulonecrotic lesions on the hands (top left and bottom)

Schematic differences between leukocytoclastic vasculitis (top right) and septic vasculitis (bottom right): the latter showing signature thrombi – the former with distinctly patent vessel lumen. Neutrophils (black dots) and karyorrhexis (tiny black dots) are present in either condition (red dots: erythrocytes)

Meningococcemia: signature fibrinoid thrombi within vessel lumina of postcapillary venules. Note paucity of inflammatory infiltrate with extremely scarce neutrophils

Leukocytoclastic vasculitis with signature **open** vascular lumen

Septic vasculitis with signature **thrombosed** vascular lumen

Figure 6.1.2 Septic Vasculitis.

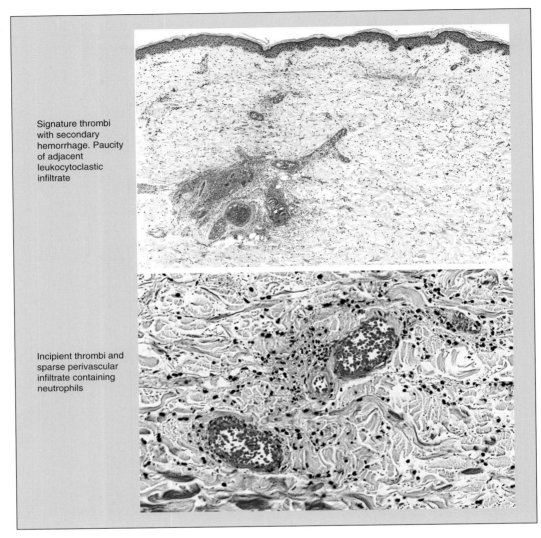

Signature thrombi with secondary hemorrhage. Paucity of adjacent leukocytoclastic infiltrate

Incipient thrombi and sparse perivascular infiltrate containing neutrophils

Figure 6.1.3 Septic Vasculitis.

In the skin, multiple microorganisms (gonococci, meningococci, staphylococci, *Pseudomonas, Aspergillus*) may induce septic vasculitis. Depending on the status of the patient's immunocompetence, clinical symptoms and course of the vasculitis may range from localized to lethal.

CF: Initially, there are widespread, mostly small erythematous, pustular, or purpuric macular lesions (petechiae), particularly at acral sites. The size and morphology of individual lesions may range from small splinter-like cutaneous hemorrhagic lesions (e.g. in gonococcemia) to large dusky-hemorrhagic and purpuric "geographic" patches and necroses (e.g. in disseminated intravascular coagulation of purpura fulminans, which is the most severe form of meningococcal sepsis).

HF:

• Fibrin thrombi within dilated postcapillary venules of the upper dermal plexus are the leading telltale sign

- The (expected) accompanying neutrophilic perivascular infiltrate may be very sparse or totally lacking (early)
- Advanced lesions present with signs of leukocytoclastic vasculitis (neutrophilic granulocytes, karyorrhexis, erythrocyte extravasation) in conjunction with obliterated vessel lumina with conspicuous thrombi (telltale sign)
- Organisms (bacteria) may be found in small clusters preferentially in the outer vessel wall or the adjacent stroma (immunohistochemistry)
- Late lesions present with epidermal involvement (neutrophilic pustules, erosions, necrosis)
- Purpura fulminans and all variants of disseminated intravascular coagulation (DIC) in the course of septic events

show massive hemorrhage, thrombi, and necrosis of adnexa and epidermis

DD: Other variants of vasculitis, purpura, and DIC.

Reference

Lipper, S., Watkins, D. L., & Kahn, L. B. (1980). Nongranulomatous septic vasculitis due to miliary tuberculosis. A pitfall in diagnosis for the pathologist. *Am J Dermatopathol*, **2**(1), 71–74.

Park, J. Y., Shin, D. H., Choi, J. S., Kim, K. H., & Bae, Y. K. (2012). Unilateral cutaneous mycotic septic vasculitis in a patient with Aspergillus vegetation in the ascending aorta. *J Dermatol*, **39**(9), 799–801.

Tomasini, C. (2015). Septic vasculitis and vasculopathy in some infectious emergencies: The perspective of the histopathologist. *G Ital Dermatol Venereol*, **150**(1), 73–85.

6.2 Bacterial Sepsis

6.2.1 Gonococcal Sepsis

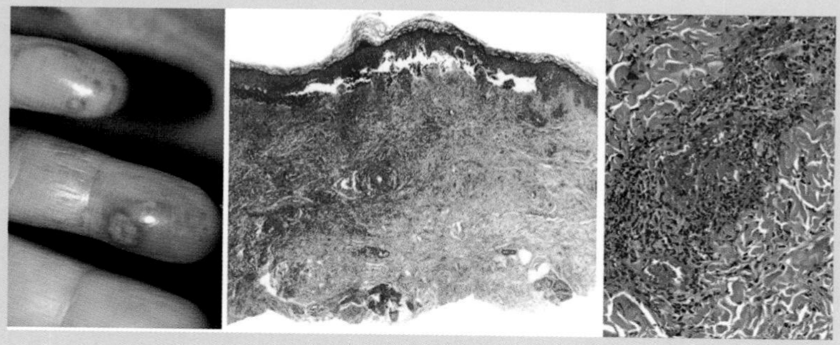

Papulopustular lesions (left and middle)

Occlusive vasculitis with neutrophils (right)

Figure 6.2.1 Variant: Gonococcal Sepsis.

Gonococcal infection may lead to hematogenous dissemination and immunoreactive septic vasculitis not only in the skin but also in other organs with arthritis and systemic clinical symptoms.

CF: Erythematous and papulopustular small lesions, preferentially on the hands and feet. Similar lesions may occur in staphylococcemia and other variants of bacterial sepsis.

HF:

- Thrombi in postcapillary venules (early)
- Thrombi in conjunction with signs of leukocytoclastic vasculitis (advanced)
- Infectious organisms usually not detectable with conventional staining methods

DD: Other types of sepsis and leukocyto-clastic vasculitis.

Reference

Bjornberg, A. (1970). Benign gonococcal sepsis. A report of 36 cases. *Acta Derm Venereol,* **50**(4), 313–316.

Shapiro, L., Teisch, J. A., & Brownstein, M. H. (1973). Dermatohistopathology of chronic gonococcal sepsis. *Arch Dermatol,* **107**(3), 403–406.

6.3 Fungal Sepsis

CF: Corresponds to other forms of sepsis.

HF:

- Diffuse dermal degeneration
- Fungal organisms both intra- and extravascular, mostly in conjunction with thrombotic vasculitis
- Tissue often replete with fungi
- Nuclear cellular debris ("dirty" dust)

DD: Other types of sepsis and of leukocytoclastic vasculitis.

Reference

Nor, N. M., & Baseri, M. M. (2015). Skin and subcutaneous infections in south-east Asia. *Curr Opin Infect Dis,* **28**(2), 133–138.

6.3.1 Variant: Penicillium Marinum Sepsis

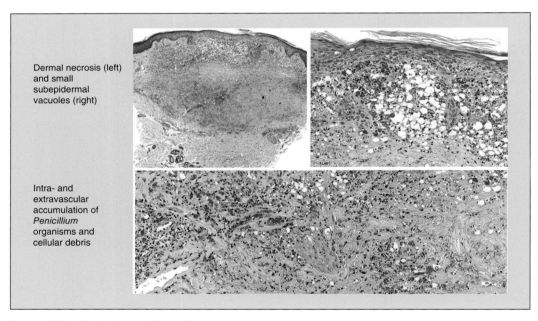

Dermal necrosis (left) and small subepidermal vacuoles (right)

Intra- and extravascular accumulation of *Penicillium* organisms and cellular debris

Figure 6.3.1 Variant: Penicillium Marinum Sepsis.

6.3.2 Variant: Candida Sepsis

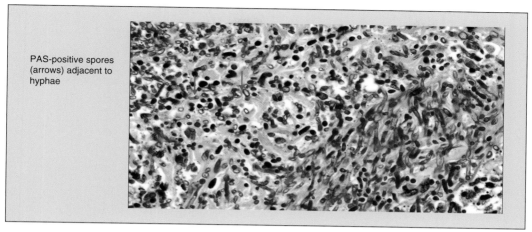

PAS-positive spores (arrows) adjacent to hyphae

Figure 6.3.2 Variant: Candida Sepsis.

6.3.3 Variant: Aspergillus Sepsis

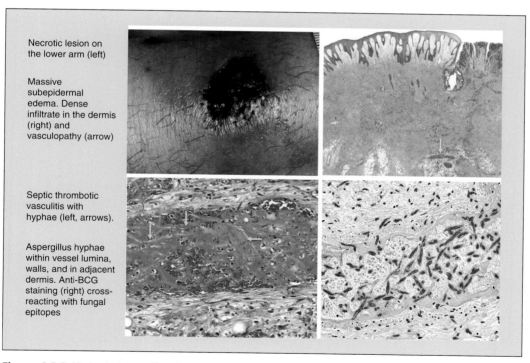

Necrotic lesion on the lower arm (left)

Massive subepidermal edema. Dense infiltrate in the dermis (right) and vasculopathy (arrow)

Septic thrombotic vasculitis with hyphae (left, arrows).

Aspergillus hyphae within vessel lumina, walls, and in adjacent dermis. Anti-BCG staining (right) cross-reacting with fungal epitopes

Figure 6.3.3 Variant: Aspergillus Sepsis.

Index

abscess 10–11
acanthamebiasis 163
acantholysis
  bacterial infections 3, 67
  viral infections 110, 112, 113, 115
acne agminata 32
acne inversa 17–18
acne papulopustulosa 7
acnitis 32
acrodermatitis chronica atrophicans 49, 56–59
  juxta-articular fibrous nodules 58–59
acrodermatitis continua suppurativa
  (Hallopeau) 72, 73
acrokeratosis verruciformis Hopf 134
acropustulosis, infantile 70
actinic reticuloid 59
actinomycosis 48–49
acute generalized exanthematous pustulosis
  (AGEP) 71–72
Aeromonas hydrophila 180
AIDS, Kaposi sarcoma 122–127
algae 107
Alternaria 103–104
amastigotes 160, 161, 162
amebiasis 163–164
Ancylostoma braziliense 174
Annelida 180
anthrax 22–23
aphthoid Pospischill–Feyrter 110
arachnids 165–170
arthropods 160, 165–172
aspergillosis 103–104
Aspergillus sepsis 187
asymmetric periflexural exanthema of
  childhood 152–153
atypical mycobacterioses 29, 39–40
Azzopardi phenomenon 145

bacillary angiomatosis 25–26
Bacillus anthracis 22
bacterial infections 1–75
  dermatoses associated with 66–67
  dermatoses mimicking 68–75
bacterial sepsis 185–186

bartonellae 25–29
Bazin's disease (erythema induratum) 38–39
BCG vaccination granuloma 30–31
bedbugs 170
bilharziasis 178–179
bird's-eye cells *see* koilocytes
black flies 176
Blastomyces dermatitidis 97
blastomycoid granuloma 98
blastomycosis 96–98
  European 94–95
  keloidal 98
  North American 96–97
  South American 101–102
blisters
  cytomegalovirus 119
  ecthyma contagiosum 149, 150
  erysipelas 14
  hand-foot-and-mouth disease 141
  herpes simplex 110
  impetigo contagiosa 3
  phlegmon 16
  septic vasculitis 182
  staphylococcal scalded skin syndrome 66, 67
  toxic epidermal necrolysis 67
  varicella zoster virus infections 112
blue cells, basophilic 136, 137
Bockhardt's ostiofolliculitis 4–5
Borrelia infections (Lyme disease) 49–59
  differential diagnosis 59
  stage I 50–54
  stage II 55–56
  stage III 56–59
botryomycosis 28–29
bowenoid papulosis 128, 135
bubo 64
bullous lesions *see* blisters
Burkitt lymphoma 117–118
Buruli ulcer 29, 47

calcified bodies 161
Calymmatobacterium granulomatis 63, 64
Candida albicans 84
Candida lipolytica 85

Atlas of Clinical Dermatopathology: Infectious and Parasitic Dermatoses, First Edition. Günter Burg,
Heinz Kutzner, Werner Kempf, Josef Feit, and Omar Sangueza.
© 2021 John Wiley & Sons Ltd. Published 2021 by John Wiley & Sons Ltd.

Candida sepsis 187
Candida tropicalis 85
candidiasis 83–85
carbuncle 12
caseating necrosis 31, 32, 35, 37
Castleman's disease, multicentric 127–128
catpox 147
cat scratch disease 25–26
cellulitis 13–15
cercariae 178–179
cercarial dermatitis 179–180
chancre, syphilitic 60–61
chancroid 63
Chicago disease 96–97
chickenpox *see* varicella
chigger itch 169
Chlamydia trachomatis 64–65
chromo(blasto)mycosis 92–93
coccidioidomycosis 100–101
conchoidal bodies 161
condylomata acuminata 128, 133
condylomata lata, verruciform 62
condylomata plana 128
corynebacteria 18–20
cowpox 147
Coxsackie virus infections 141–142
creeping eruption 174
crusted scabies 167, 168
cryptococcosis 94–95
Cryptococcus gattii 95
Cryptococcus neoformans 95, 97
cysticercosis 177
cytomegalovirus 119–120

Darier's disease 134
deer pox 147
dematiaceous organisms 106
Demodex folliculorum mites 166
dermatitis exfoliativa neonatorum 66–67
dermatitis verrucosa 92–93
dermatophytes 78, 79–81
desert fever 100–101
disseminated intravascular coagulation (DIC) 185
Donovan bodies 63, 64
donovanosis 63–64
Duran-Nicolas-Favre disease 64–65

eccrine hidradenitis, mitoxantrone-associated localized
    neutrophilic 73–74
ecthyma contagiosum 9, 149–150
ecthyma gangrenosum 9–10
ecthyma simplex 9
ectoparasites 160, 165–172, 180
eczema herpeticum 110
elephantiasis 64, 175
emmonsiosis 102–103
Entamoeba histolytica 163–164

enterovirus 71: 141
epidermodysplasia verruciformis 128, 136–137
Epstein–Barr virus (EBV) 117–119
erosive pustular dermatitis, scalp 74–75
eruptive pseudoangiomatosis 153–154
erysipelas 13–15
erysipeloid 21–22
erythema induratum Bazin (EIB) 38–39
erythema infectiosum 139
erythema (chronicum) migrans 49, 50–51
erythema necroticans 46–47
erythema nodosum leprosum (ENL) 46–47
erythrasma 18–19
erythrophagocytosis 124, 163, 164
European blastomycosis 94–95
exanthema subitum 120

facies leonina 43, 44
fifth disease 139
filariasis 175
fish eye cells 119
fish tank mycobacteriosis 29, 39–40
Fite-Faraco stain 40, 44, 45
foamy cells 45, 46, 47
follicular spicules of nose, multiple sclerosis 143
folliculitis
    Bockhardt 4–5
    deep 11–12
    Demodex 166
    differential diagnosis 7–8
    Malassezia (Pityrosporum) 87–88
    necrotizing zoster 115
    Pseudomonas 5–6
    superficial 4–6
fungal infections 77–107
    opportunistic 103–107
    subcutaneous 90–93
    superficial cutaneous 78–90
    systemic (deep) 93–103
fungal sepsis 186–187
furuncle 11–12
Fusarium 105

Gianotti–Crosti syndrome 154–155
gloves-and-socks syndrome 140
gnathostoma 166
gonococcal sepsis 185–186
gonorrhea 59–60
Gram-negative folliculitis 5–6
granuloma inguinale (venereum) 63–64
granuloma pyogenicum 28–29
granuloma trichophyticum 82–83
Guarnieri bodies 149, 150
gummatous lesions 62

Haemophilus ducreyi 63
hairy leukoplakia 118–119

hand-foot-and-mouth disease   141–142
Hansen disease *see* leprosy
harvest mites   169
Heck's disease (morbus Heck)   128
helminthic infections   173–180
herpes simplex (HSV-1, HSV-2)   110–111, 112
herpes viruses   110–128
herpes zoster   111, 112, 113–117
    associated vasculitis   116
    folliculitis, necrotizing   115
    postherpetic reactions   117
hidradenitis, mitoxantrone-associated neutrophilic
        eccrine localized   73–74
hidradenitis suppurativa   17–18
Hirudinea   180
Hirudo medicinalis   180
histoid leprosy (HL)   45
histoplasmosis   99–100
hookworms, larva migrans   174
Hortaea werneckii   89
hot tub dermatitis   5–6
human herpes virus 3 (HHV-3) *see* varicella zoster virus
human herpes virus 4 (HHV-4)   117–119
human herpes virus 5 (HHV-5)   119–120
human herpes virus 6 (HHV-6)   120
human herpes virus 7 (HHV-7)   121–122
human herpes virus 8 (HHV-8)   122–128
human herpes virus (HHV) infections   110–128
human papilloma virus (HPV) infections   128–137
hyaline globules   124, 126
hyalohyphomycoses   105
hyperhidrosis   19, 20
hyperpigmentation   89
hypostome   51, 170

impetigo contagiosa   2–3
Indian file-like infiltrates   9, 51, 53
infantile acropustulosis   70
insects   170–172
invisible dermatosis   86, 87
Ixodes ticks   49, 50

juxta-articular fibrous nodules, acrodermatitis chronica
        atrophicans   58–59

Kaposi sarcoma   122–127
    classic Mediterranean   126
    immunodeficiency-associated   126
    lymphangioma-like pattern   125, 126
    macular (patch) stage   122, 126
    plaque stage   123, 126
    tumor/nodular stage   124, 126
Kaposi's varicelliform eruption   110
keloidal blastomycosis   98
keratoma sulcatum   19
Klebsiella (Calymmatobacterium) granulomatis   63, 64
Klebsiella pneumoniae rhinoscleromatis   24

koilocytes   130, 131, 132, 133
Koplik spots   138

Lacazia loboi   98
Langhans giant cells
    fish tank granuloma   39, 40
    leprosy   41, 43
    lobomycosis   98
    tuberculosis   35, 36, 37
larva currens   174
larva migrans   174
larynx papilloma   128
leeches   180
Leishmania mexicana   162
leishmaniasis   160–162
leonine facies   43, 44
lepromatous leprosy   43–44
leprosy   40–47
    borderline   42–43
    classification   40
    lepromatous   43–44
    tuberculoid   41–42
    variants   45–47
leukocytoclastic vasculitis
    acute generalized exanthematous pustulosis   72
    herpes simplex   111
    herpes zoster   114, 116
    insect bites   170
    Mediterranean tick fever   66
    septic vasculitis   183, 185
Lewandowsky–Lutz dysplasia *see* epidermodysplasia
        verruciformis
lichen scrofulosorum   36
lilac ring   55
Loa loa   175
Lobo disease   98
lobomycosis   98
lobular capillary hemangioma   28–29
localized neutrophilic eccrine hidradenitis,
        mitoxantrone-associated   73–74
Lucio phenomenon   46–47
lupus miliaris disseminatus faciei (LMDF)   31–32
lupus verrucosa   34
lupus vulgaris (LV)   32–36
Lyme disease *see* Borrelia infections
lymphadenosis cutis benigna   51, 52–54
lymphocytoma cutis   51, 52–54
lymphogranuloma inguinale (venereum)   64–65
lymphoma, Burkitt   117–118

Madura foot   91
Majocchi's granuloma   82–83
Malassezia (Pityrosporum) folliculitis   87–88
Malassezia furfur   86, 88
Mantoux test   33
measles   138–139
Mediterranean tick fever   66

Medlar bodies 93

meningococcemia 183

mercury 71

Merkel cell carcinoma 144–145

Merkel cell polyomavirus 145

Michaelis-Gutmann bodies 161

Mikulicz cells 24, 25

milker's nodule 150–151

mites 165–169

mitoxantrone-associated localized neutrophilic eccrine
    hidradenitis 73–74

molds 78

molluscum bodies 151, 152

molluscum contagiosum 151–152

moniliasis 83–84

monkey pox 146, 149

morbus Heck 128

morphea 55–56

mosquitoes 170, 175

mucormycosis 104–105

multiple sclerosis, follicular spicules of nose 143

mycetoma 91

mycobacterial infections 29–47

Mycobacterium kansasii 29

Mycobacterium leprae 40

Mycobacterium marinum 29, 40

Mycobacterium tuberculosis 30, 33

Mycobacterium ulcerans 29, 47

mycoses *see* fungal infections

mycosis fungoides-like borreliosis 57–58

myiasis 170

Nazzaro syndrome 143

necrotizing fasciitis 17

necrotizing (herpes) zoster 111

necrotizing (herpes) zoster folliculitis 115

neuroendocrine carcinoma of skin, primary,
    144–145

neuts in the horn 80

nocardiosis 23

North American blastomycosis 96–97

Norwegian scabies 167, 168

onchocerciasis 176

opportunistic fungal infections 103–107

orf 9, 149–150

Oroya fever 27

orthopox virus infections 146–149

ostiofolliculitis (Bockhardt) 4–5

owl's eye cells 119, 120

panniculitis 38

papular purpuric gloves-and-socks
    syndrome 140

papulonecrotic tuberculid 37

paracoccidioidomycosis 101–102

paralysis, progressive 62

parapox virus infections 149–152

parasitoses 159–172, 173–180

paraviral exanthems 152–157

parvovirus infections 139–140

pediculi 170

pemphigus neonatorum 66–67

Penicillium marinum sepsis 186

perianal streptococcal dermatitis 6

periflexural exanthema of childhood,
    asymmetric 152–153

phaeohyphomycosis 106

Phlebotomus sand flies 161

phlegmon 15–16

phycomycosis 104–105

piedra 90

Piedraia hortae 90

pitted keratolysis 19

pityriasis lichenoides 155–157

pityriasis lichenoides chronica (PLC) 156

pityriasis lichenoides et varioliformis acuta
    (PLEVA) 156, 157

pityriasis rosea 121–122

pityriasis (tinea) versicolor 86–87

Pityrosporum (Malassezia) folliculitis 87–88

Pityrosporum ovale or *orbiculare* 86

plantar warts (verrucae plantaris) 128, 131

plumber's itch 174

polyoma virus infections 142–145

postherpetic cutaneous reactions 117

poxviruses 146–152

promontory sign 123, 126

protothecosis, cutaneous 107

protozoan diseases 160–165

psammoma bodies 161

Pseudallescheria boydii 105

pseudofolliculitis barbae 8

pseudolymphoma 52–54

Pseudomonas folliculitis 5–6

pseudo-rosette pattern 50, 51

psoriasis pustulosa 72–73

purpura fulminans 185

pustula maligna 22

pustular ulcerative dermatosis, scalp 74–75

pyoderma gangrenosum 68–69

pyogenic granuloma 28–29

Q-fever 65

rhinoscleroma 24–25

rhinosporidiosis 164–165

rickettsial infections 65–66

ringed worms 180

ringworm *see* dermatophytes

Ritter disease 66–67

river blindness 176

Rocha–Lima bodies 27

Rochalimaea 25–29

roseola infantum 120

Russell bodies 24, 25

sand flea   171–172
San Joaquin fever   100–101
scabies   167–168
scabies crustosa (Norwegian scabies)   167, 168
scabies granuloma   168
scalp, erosive pustular dermatitis   74–75
Schaumann bodies   161
schistosomiasis   178–179
scleroderma-like lesions   55–56
scrofuloderma   35–36
scybala   167, 168
seborrheic dermatitis   88–89
segmented worms   180
sepsis   181–187
   bacterial   185–186
   fungal   186–187
septic vasculitis   182–185
   Aspergillus sepsis   187
   ecthyma gangrenosum   9, 10
   gonococcal sepsis   185
sexually transmitted infections   59–65
shingles *see* herpes zoster
sixth disease   120
slapped cheek disease   139
smallpox   148–149
South American blastomycosis   101–102
sparganosis   177–178
spider bites   169
Splendore–Hoeppli phenomenon   23
spongiform pustulation   72, 73
sporotrichosis   90–91
staphylococcal infections   2–18
staphylococcal Lyell syndrome   66–67
staphylococcal scalded skin syndrome   66–67
starry sky pattern   118
steel-gray nuclei   110, 112, 113
steering wheel pattern   101, 102
streptococcal gangrene   17
streptococcal infections   2–18
Strongyloides stercoralis   174
sulfur granules   48, 49
Sweet syndrome   69
swimmers' itch   179–180
swimming pool mycobacteriosis   29, 39–40
syphilis   60–62
   stage I, 60–61
   stage II, 61–62
   stage III, 62

tabes dorsalis   62
Taenia solium   177
thrombi   183, 184, 185
ticks   170
   Lyme disease   49, 50, 51
   rickettsial diseases   65
tinea   78, 79–81
tinea amiantacea   79
tinea barbae   80–81

tinea capitis   80–81
tinea corporis   79–80
tinea faciei   79–80
tinea favosa   81
tinea nigra   89
tinea profunda   80
tinea (pityriasis) versicolor   86–87
tingible body macrophages   53, 54
torulosis   94–95
toxic epidermal necrolysis   67
trabecular carcinoma of Toker   144–145
Treponema pallidum   60–62
trichobacteriosis (trichomycosis) palmellina   20
Trichobilharzia   179
trichodysplasia spinulosa   142–143
trichomycosis nodosa alba and nigra   90
Trichophyton schoenleinii   81
Trichosporon asahii   90
tricolore sign   149, 150
trombidiosis   169
trophozoites   163, 164
tuberculoid leprosy   41–42
tuberculosis cutis   29–39
   primary   30
   variants   34–36
tuberculosis cutis colliquativa   35–36
tuberculosis cutis lichenoides   36
tuberculosis cutis verrucosa   34
tungiasis   171–172

ulceration
   Buruli ulcer   47
   coccidioidomycosis   100
   ecthyma gangrenosum   9
   emmonsiosis   102
   Entamoeba histolytica   163
   erosive pustular dermatitis of the scalp   75
   leishmaniasis   160, 161
   paracoccidioidomycosis   101
   phaeohyphomycosis   106
   pyoderma gangrenosum   68, 69
   venereal disease   60, 63, 64
ulcus molle   63

vaccinia inoculata   148
valley fever   100–101
varicella   111, 112–113, 114
varicella zoster virus (VZV) infections   111–117
variola vera   148–149
vasculitis
   erythema nodosum leprosum   46–47
   herpes simplex   110–111
   leukocytoclastic *see* leukocytoclastic vasculitis
   pyoderma gangrenosum   68, 69
   rickettsial infections   65, 66
   septic *see* septic vasculitis
   zoster-associated   116
venereal diseases   59–65

verrucae planae   128, 132–133
verruca plantaris   128, 131
verruca vulgaris   128, 129–131
verruciform condylomata lata   62
verrucosis generalisata   136–137
verruga peruana   27
viral exanthema   137–139
viral infections   109–157
Virchow cells   43, 44
von Rittershain disease   66–67

Warthin–Finkeldey cells   128, 139
warts   128–133

whirlpool dermatitis   5–6
worms, parasitic   173–180
Wuchereria bancrofti   175

yeasts   78

zoster-associated vasculitis   116
zoster folliculitis, necrotizing   115
zoster incognito   115
zygomycosis   104–105